Clinical Cases in Dermatology

Series Editor
Robert A. Norman, Tampa, FL, USA

This series of concise practical guides is designed to facilitate the clinical decision-making process by reviewing a number of cases and defining the various diagnostic and management decisions open to clinicians.

Each title is illustrated and diverse in scope, enabling the reader to obtain relevant clinical information regarding both standard and unusual cases in a rapid, easy to digest format. Each focuses on one disease or patient group, and includes common cases to allow readers to know they are doing things right if they follow the case guidelines.

Torello M. Lotti • Mohammad Jafferany
Xing-Hua Gao • Ayman Abdelmaksoud
Editors

Clinical Cases in Facial Erythema

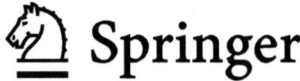 Springer

Editors
Torello M. Lotti
Dermatology
Marconi University
Rome, Roma, Italy

Xing-Hua Gao
Department of Dermatology
First Hospital of China Medical University
Shenyang, Liaoning, China

Mohammad Jafferany
Psychodermatology, Psychiatry &
Behavioral Sciences
Central Michigan University
College of Medicine
Saginaw, MI, USA

Ayman Abdelmaksoud
Mansoura Dermatology, Venererology,
and Leprology Hospital
Mansoura, Egypt

ISSN 2730-6178   ISSN 2730-6186   (electronic)
Clinical Cases in Dermatology
ISBN 978-3-031-05995-7   ISBN 978-3-031-05996-4   (eBook)
https://doi.org/10.1007/978-3-031-05996-4

This Springer imprint is published by the registered company Springer Nature Switzerland AG
The registered company address is: Gewerbestrasse 11, 6330 Cham, Switzerland

Contents

1   **55-Year-Old Woman with Redness on Face and Stiffness in Hand** . .   1
Abdullah Demirbaş and Mehmet Akyürek

2   **59-Year-Old Woman with Redness on Face and Edema**   5
Işıl Göğem İmren, Selami Aykut Temiz, Erdem Çomut,
Şule Gökşin, and Şeniz Duygulu

3   **A 55-Year-Old Female with Bilateral Malar Fixed
Erythema and Periorbital Edema**   9
Zuhal Metin and Koray Durmaz

4   **A Case of Stubborn Facial Redness**   15
Sabha Mushtaq

5   **A Female in Middle Age with Red Nodule**   19
Runping Fang, Lu Wang, Rongming Yang, Shuanglin Li,
and Yuan Li

6   **A Female with Erythema and Telangiectasis**   25
Ling Yu, Jian-Bo Wang, Shu-Zhen Zhang, and Shou-Min Zhang

7   **A Female with Nodules**   29
Yining Wang and Xing-Hua Gao

8   **A Female with Thick Crust on Lip**   33
Jing Lan, Wei Huo, Hao Guo, Qian An, and Xing-Hua Gao

9   **A Middle-Aged Male with Multiple Plaques**   37
Xi Wang and Songmei Geng

10   **A Middle-Aged Man Presenting with a New Asymmetrical
Poikilodematous Erythema on the Lateral Neck**   41
Paweł Pietkiewicz

11 **A Middle-Aged Man with Erythema and
Nodules on His Face**   45
Runping Fang

12 **A Red Signal for Cancer**   51
Ratnakar Shukla, Sharmila Patil, Aswathy Radhakrishan,
and Anant Patil

13 **A Woman with Facial Butterfly Erythema**   57
Wen-Jia Yang, Hao Guo, Tian-Hua Xu, Xing-Hua Gao,
and Jiu-Hong Li

14 **An Elderly Female with Lacy, Reticulated and
White Streaks**   61
Bing-Yan Yang, Nan Yu, and Yong-Long Gao

15 **An Intriguing Case of Red Face**   63
Elena Mirceska Arsovska and Katerina Damevska

16 **An Old Women with Erythema, Pimples and Pain over
Neck, Waist and Abdomen**   69
Xiao-Dong Li, Juan Chen, Hao Guo, and Xing-Hua Gao

17 **Asymptomatic Erythematous Discoloration**   75
Katerina Damevska and Stefana Damevska

18 **Bilateral Periorbital Erythema**   81
Hadir Shakshouk and Julia S. Lehman

19 **Cutaneous Angiosarcoma on Scalp and Face in an
Elderly Patient**   85
Jin-Fa Dou, Jian-Bo Wang, Hui Li, Yu-Ping Wang,
and Shou-Min Zhang

20 **Disseminated Vesicular Lesions in an
Immunocompetent Individual**   89
Shashank Bhargava and George Kroumpouzos

21 **Erythematous Papular Lesions of the Face**   95
Erdal Polat, Muazzez Cigdem Oba, and Zekayi Kutlubay

22 **Facial Erythema and Flushing in a 55-Year-Old Female**   99
Tugba Kevser Uzuncakmak and Zekayi Kutlubay

23 **Generalised Exfoliating "Figurate Erythema":
A Rare Cause**   105
Lawrence Chukwudi Nwabudike and Alin Laurentiu Tatu

24 **Numerous Nodules on the Forehead**   111
Qu Qi and Xing-Hua Gao

25 **One Patient with Facial Tan Patches** 115
    Ya-Ning Jiao, Nan Yu, Xin-Hong Ge, Li Xia, Yuan-Yuan Shang,
    and Ke-Xin Li

26 **Red Face in a 57-Year-Old Patient with Pulmonary Cancer** 119
    Selami Aykut Temiz and Recep Dursun

27 **Red Facial Patches on the Forehead** 123
    Uwe Wollina

28 **Red-Purple Plaque on the Right Side of the Neck** 127
    Filippo Viviani, Alba Guglielmo, Carlotta Baraldi, Federica Filippi,
    Alessandro Pileri, and Federico Bardazzi

29 **Ulcero-Crusted Lesions of the Face** 131
    Diego Abbenante, Miriam Anna Carpanese, Michelangelo La Placa,
    and Federico Bardazzi

30 **Unilateral Erythema** 135
    Monika Fida, Ritjana Mala, and Oljeda Kaçani

Index 139

Chapter 1
55-Year-Old Woman with Redness on Face and Stiffness in Hand

Abdullah Demirbaş and Mehmet Akyürek

A 55-year-old female with autoimmune hypothyroidism and Sjogren's disease, applied to the Dermatology clinic with redness on her face. In addition, the patient has complaints of purpleness, redness, and pallor in her hands dependent on weather changes. The patient had a history of 2 months with initially mild but progressively increased. The patient had no any other symptoms, but she stated that exposure to sun increases her complaints. Physical examination revealed diffuse erythema and telangiectasia in both the malar and nasal regions, and mild sclerosis and pallor in the hands (Figs. 1.1 and 1.2). Since patient had a rheumatologic disease and describes Raynaud's phenomenon, capilleroscopy was performed to the fingers using computed dermatoscopy. In capillaroscopy, capillaries were detected as dilated and tortuous. In laboratory examinations there were increased sedimentation and Anti-nuclear antibody (ANA), anti-RO52, anti-SS-A, anti-Ribonucleoprotein (anti-RNP), anti-SM positivity. In thorax tomography esophagus was detected as dilated (Fig. 1.3).

Based on the Case Description and the Photograph, What Is Your Diagnosis?

Rosacea (Erythematotelangiectatic type)
   Systemic lupus erythematosus
   CREST Syndrome (limited systemic scleroderma)

A. Demirbaş (✉)
Department of Dermatology, Kocaeli University, Faculty of Medicine, Kocaeli, Turkey
e-mail: abdullah.demirbas@kocaeli.edu.tr

M. Akyürek
Faculty of Medicine, Department of Dermatology, Selcuk University, Konya, Turkey

© The Author(s), under exclusive license to Springer Nature Switzerland AG 2022
T. M. Lotti et al. (eds.), *Clinical Cases in Facial Erythema*, Clinical Cases in Dermatology, https://doi.org/10.1007/978-3-031-05996-4_1

Fig. 1.1 Erythema and
telangiectasia in both the
malar and nasal regions

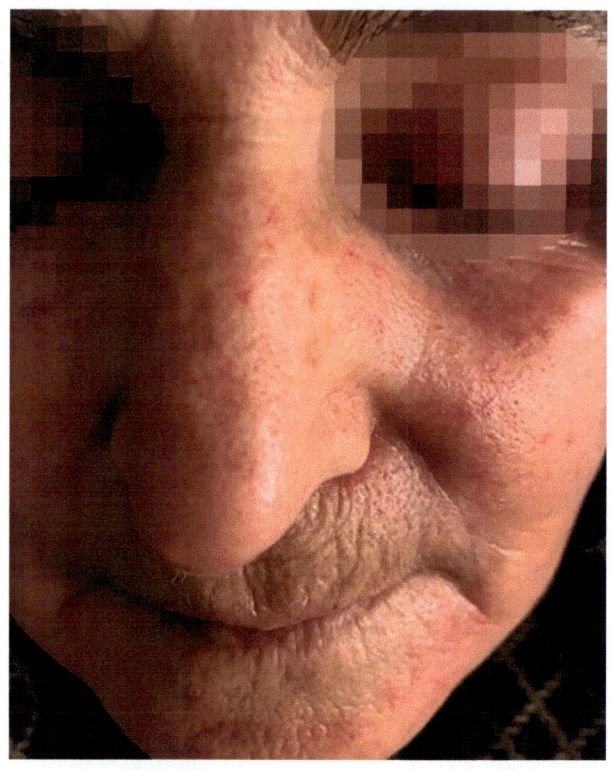

Fig. 1.2 Stiffness and
pallor in hands

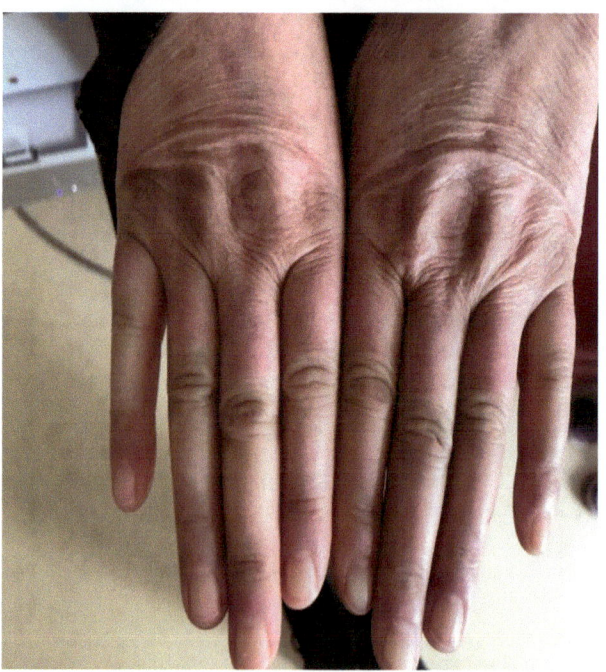

Fig. 1.3 Dilated
esophagus (white arrow)

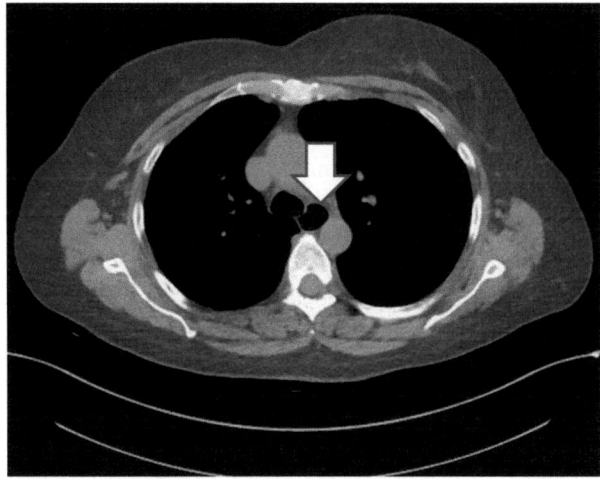

Diagnosis

CREST Syndrome

Systemic sclerosis is a rare chronic auto-inflammatory disease. Its etiopathogenesis is not fully known. The vascular changes, autoimmune mechanisms and tissue fibrosis evolve with the effect of genetic and environmental factors. Two types have been defined; localized and systemic. Morphea is localized form of scleroderma and affects only the skin. Systemic sclerosis is divided into two main types; limited and diffuse. CREST syndrome is assumed subtype of limited scleroderma, composed of calcinosis, Raynaud's phenomenon, esophageal dysmotility, sclerodactyly, and telangiectasia. The diagnosis is made by having three or more criteria. Anti-nuclear antibody (ANA), Anti-centromere, Anti-SCL70, Anti-RNA polymerase III positivity can be also detected. Pulmonary or renal involvement, pulmonary hypertension, pericarditis, pericardial effusion, arrhythmias, arthritis, arthralgia, myalgia, hypothyroidism and autoimmune thyroid disorders, and Sjogren's disease may accompany CREST Syndrome as well as diffuse scleroderma [1, 2].

Rosacea is a common, chronic, inflammatory disease that involves central part of the face. It is characterized by erythema, telangiectasia, papules, pustules, fibrosis, and deformities. There are four different clinical types of rosacea: erythematotelangiectatic, papulopustular, phymatous, and ocular. Erythematolegiectatic subtype of rosacea is characterized by transient or persistent central erythema and telangiectasias. Symptoms of erythematolegiectatic type include burning, stinging, and itching [3]. Although pathogenesis of the disease has not been fully elucidated, several studies have demonstrated the roles of abnormal activations of Th-1 and Th-17 cells and cathelicidins. Triggering factors such as ultraviolet light, temperature changes, alcohol, and spicy foods can activate the cathelicidin–LL 37 signaling pathway and pro-inflammatory cytokines such as IL-1, IL-6, IL-8, TNF-α, IFN-γ, IL-17A, and IL-22 through Th 1 and Th 17 pathways. The diagnosis is usually made clinically [4].

Systemic lupus erythematosus is a chronic, progressive, heterogeneous auto-immune disease. It generally seen in young women and can affects many organs as a systemic disease. Although the etiology is unclear, drugs, diet, hormones, stress, sun exposure, smoking, and genetic predisposition are the most blamed causes. The abnormal activation of the immune mechanism triggered by etiological factors causes multiple organ damage. The most commonly reported symptoms and clinical signs are fever, fatigue, loss of appetite, weight loss, photosensitivity, discoid or malar rash, alopecia, aphthous ulcers, periungal erythema, splinter hemorrhages, kidney glomerulonephritis or nephrotic syndrome, myalgia, arthritis, arthralgia, pericarditis, pericardial effusion, pleuritis, neuropsychiatric disorders. In laboratory findings, anti-nuclear antibodies (ANA), anti-RNP, anti-SM, dsDNA positivity, and low complement can be seen [5].

Key Points
1. The subtype of limited scleroderma is known to be CREST syndrome.
2. CREST syndrome is composed of calcinosis, Raynaud's phenomenon, esopha-geal dysmotility, sclerodactyly, and telangiectasia.
3. The diagnosis is made by having three or more criteria.
4. Capillaroscopy is useful in the diagnosis of CREST syndrome.

References

1. Adigun R, Goyal A, Bansal P, Hariz A. Systemic Sclerosis. 2020 Aug 10. In: StatPearls [Internet]. Treasure Island (FL): StatPearls Publishing; 2020.
2. Zulian F. New developments in localized scleroderma. Curr Opin Rheumatol. 2008;20(5):601–7. https://doi.org/10.1097/BOR.0b013e328309a5eb.
3. Rainer BM, Kang S, Chien AL. Rosacea: epidemiology, pathogenesis, and treatment. Dermatoendocrinol. 2017;9(1):e1361574. https://doi.org/10.1080/19381980.2017.1361574.
4. Steinhoff M, Buddenkotte J, Aubert J, Sulk M, Novak P, Schwab VD, Mess C, Cevikbas F, Rivier M, Carlavan I, Déret S, Rosignoli C, Metze D, Luger TA, Voegel JJ. Clinical, cellular, and molecular aspects in the pathophysiology of rosacea. J Investig Dermatol Symp Proc. 2011;15(1):2–11. https://doi.org/10.1038/jidsymp.2011.7.
5. Gurevitz SL, Snyder JA, Wessel EK, Frey J, Williamson BA. Systemic lupus erythematosus: a review of the disease and treatment options. Consult Pharm. 2013;28(2):110–21. https://doi.org/10.4140/TCP.n.2013.110.

Chapter 2
59-Year-Old Woman with Redness on Face and Edema

Işıl Göğem İmren, Selami Aykut Temiz, Erdem Çomut, Şule Gökşin, and Şeniz Duygulu

A 59-year-old woman presents with a 3-month history of gradually enlargement of axillary and cervical lympnode and reddening of skin prominently on face (Fig. 2.1), proximal trunk. Patient stated that, swelling of scalp and serious discharge on her ears gradually increase during the last 1 month. Dermatologic examination showed the erythematous skin of the scalp and glabella was thrown into cerebriform folds.

General examination revealed multiple, enlarged, non-tender, discrete, mobile lymphnodes in bilateral cervical, axillary regions, the largest of which was 5 cm × 6 cm in the right axillary region, associated with hepatosplenomegaly. On hematological examination, leukocytosis (42.4 × 109/L) and an increased serum lactatede hydrogenase level was detected.

Histopathological examination was performed from the cutaneous biopsy taken for differential diagnosis (Figs. 2.2 and 2.3). Cutaneous biopsy sections revealed infiltration of large, irregular polygonal cells arranged in cohesive sheets extending throughout the dermis. Neoplastic lymphoid cells expressed CD3, CD4, CD30 and were negative for CD20, CD8 and MUM1. Then, lymphnode biopsy sections revealed infiltration of large, irregular polygonal cells arranged in cohesive sheets extending perinodal fibroadipous tissue. Neoplastic lymphoid cells in the lymphnode sections expressed CD3, CD4, CD30, CD5, CD7, CD2, MUM1, granzyme B and were negative for CD20, PAX5, CD8, ALK and EBV (EBV-encoded small RNA). Finally, the diagnosis was made as ALK-negative anaplastic large cell lymphoma.

I. G. İmren (✉) · Ş. Gökşin · Ş. Duygulu
Department of Dermatology, Pamukkale University, School of Medicine, Denizli, Turkey

S. A. Temiz
Clinic of Dermatology, Konya Ereğli State Hospital, Konya, Turkey

E. Çomut
Department of Pathology, Pamukkale University, School of Medicine, Denizli, Turkey

Fig. 2.1 Widespread redness and edema on the face, as well as enlarged skin sulci

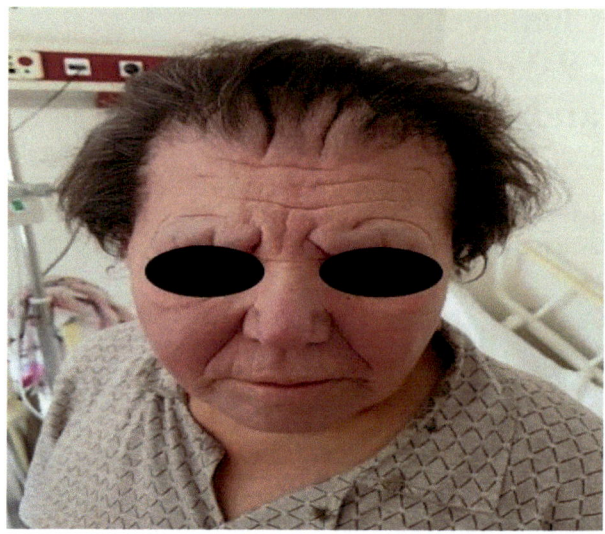

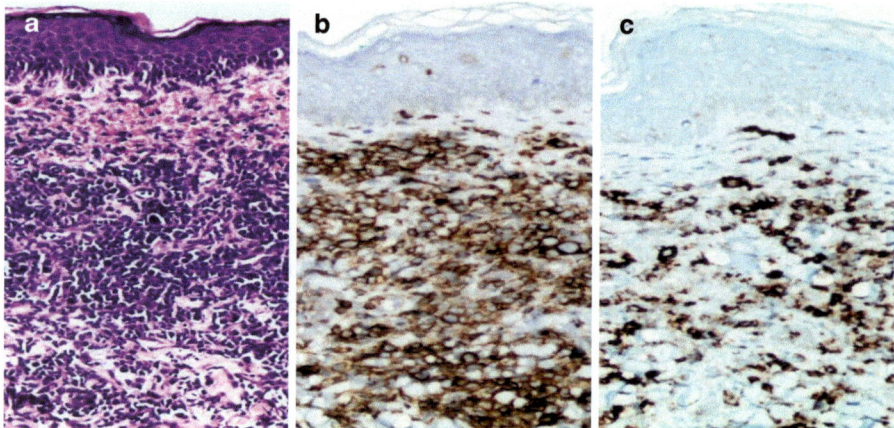

Fig. 2.2 (**a**) Anaplastic large cell lymphoma infiltrates the dermis in sheets of anaplastic cells. Note that the tumor does not show epidermotropism (H&E, ×200). (**b**) Diffuse membranous positivity with CD4 in tumor cells (×200). (**c**) Membranous positivity with CD30 in anaplastic tumor cells (×200)

What Is Your Diagnosis Based on the Case Description and the Photos?

- CD30 positive lymphoproliferative disease
- Mikozis Fungoides
- Primary İdiopatic Cutis Verticis Gyrata
- Cutis Verticis Gyrata secondary to malign infiltration

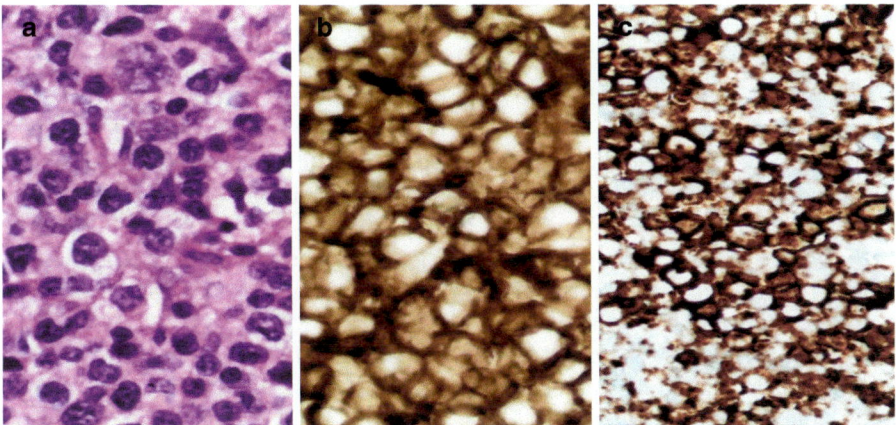

Fig. 2.3 (a) Diffuse infiltration of large tumor cells with pleomorphic nuclei in the lymph node. (H&E, ×400). (b) Diffuse membranous positivity with CD4 in tumor cells (×400). (c) Diffuse membranous positivity with CD30 in anaplastic tumor cells (×400)

Diagnosis

ALK-negative anaplastic large cell lymphoma.
   Cutis Verticis Gyrata secondary to malign infiltration.

Discussion

The primary form of cutis verticis gyrata, that is characterized by abnormal histology of the skin, is further divided based on the absence or presence of underlying neuro-ophthalmological manifestations into essential and non-essential respectively [1]. Secondary cutis verticis gyrata has been reported to occur secondary to endocrine diseases, infections, hereditary disorders, inflammatory dermatosis, benign and malignant tumors [2]. Secondary cutis verticis gyrata is considered to be a symptom of a variety of underlying causes, and in this case the pathophysiology may be associated with the specific underlying condition [3]. Histopathological examination of the cutaneous biopsy taken from our case also indicated ALK-negative anaplastic large cell lymphoma cutaneous infiltration. When the literature is reviewed, cases of secondary cutis verticis gyrata due to systemic T-cell lymphoma [4] were reported due to acute monoblastic leukemia [5] in one case. There has been no case of secondary cutis verticis gyrata due to ALK-negative anaplastic large cell lymphoma in the literature.
   Cutis verticis gyrata is characterized by symmetrical, excessive scalp folds with deep grooves and folds. Hypertrophy and folding of the skin creates an appearance that mimics the appearance of the cerebral gyrus [6]. Erythema is more pronounced

when edema in the cutis verticis gyrata is outside of the scalp (for example, on the forehead) [6]. Therefore, it should be expected to cause a red face in the case of facial involvement as in our case.

Key Points
- Secondary cutis verticis gyrata has been reported to occur secondary to endocrine diseases, infections, hereditary disorders, inflammatory dermatosis, benign and malignant tumors
- Secondary cutis verticis gyrata is considered to be a symptom of a variety of underlying causes, and in this case the pathophysiology may be associated with the specific underlying condition
- Erythema is more pronounced when edema in the cutis verticis gyrata is outside of the scalp, therefore, it should be expected to cause a red face in the case of facial involvement as in our case.

References

1. Dumas P, Medard de Chardon V, Balaguer T, et al. Primary essential cutis verticis gyrata: case report and literature review. Ann Chir Plast Esthet. 2010;55:243–8.
2. Larsen F, Birchall N. Cutis verticis gyrata: three cases with different aetiologies that demonstrate the classification system. Australas J Dermatol. 2007;48(2):91–4.
3. Ulrich J, Franke I, Gollnick H. Cutis verticis gyrata secondary to acne scleroticans capitis. J Eur Acad Dermatol Venereol. 2004;18(4):499–502.
4. George A, George L, Mahabal G, Bindra M, Pulimood S. Systemic T cell lymphoma presenting as cutis verticis gyrata. Indian J Dermatol Venereol Leprol. 2015;81(6).
5. Passarini B, Neri IRIA, Patrizi A, Masina M. Cutis verticis gyrata secondary to acute monoblastic leukemia. Acta Derm Venereol. 1993;73(2):148–9.
6. Jung JS, Lim NK. A rare case of secondary cutis verticis gyrata on the forehead. J Wound Manage Res. 2020;16(2):113–6.

Chapter 3
A 55-Year-Old Female with Bilateral Malar Fixed Erythema and Periorbital Edema

Zuhal Metin and Koray Durmaz

Case Report

A 55-year-old woman, with no personal or family medical history, presented with a 3-year history of redness, itching, burning, and tenderness on the center of the face. She had also involuntary weight loss for 3 months. Previously, in the beginning of symptoms, she had unprotected UV exposure during summer months. At that time, redness and itching also occurred in her forearms. A biopsy had been performed from the erythematous area on the right forearm confirmed the diagnosis of polymorphous light eruption (PLE) in the outer center. The pathologic findings were mild hyperkeratosis, epidermal spongiosis, Perivascular lymphohistiocytic infiltrate in superficial dermis and degeneration of elastic fibers. When the patient applied to us, there was no rash in her arms (Fig. 3.1) however, fixed erythema in the bilateral malar areas of the face and edema on the eyelids (Fig. 3.2). The patient had no history of contact sensitization.

Standardized skin surface biopsy (SSSB) procedure was performed from the right cheek and demodex density was observed 20 per cm^2 in the microscopy. She was administered several tests include biopsy with hematoxylin-eosin (H&E) stain and the results was:

- Cell blood count was normal RBC: 5.12 T/l, WBC: 7.52 G/l, PLT: 310 T/l
- Cancer antigen 15–3 (CA 15–3) was mild high: 33.2 U/mL
- Thyroid microsomal antibody (TMAB) was positive.
- BI-RADS 1 was revealed at mammogram.

Z. Metin
Department of Dermatology, Kirsehir Ahi Evran University, Kirsehir, Turkey

K. Durmaz (✉)
Department of Dermatology, Yasam Hospital, Kirikkale, Turkey

© The Author(s), under exclusive license to Springer Nature   9
Switzerland AG 2022
T. M. Lotti et al. (eds.), *Clinical Cases in Facial Erythema*, Clinical Cases in
Dermatology, https://doi.org/10.1007/978-3-031-05996-4_3

Fig. 3.1 Bilateral
forearms were normal
appearance

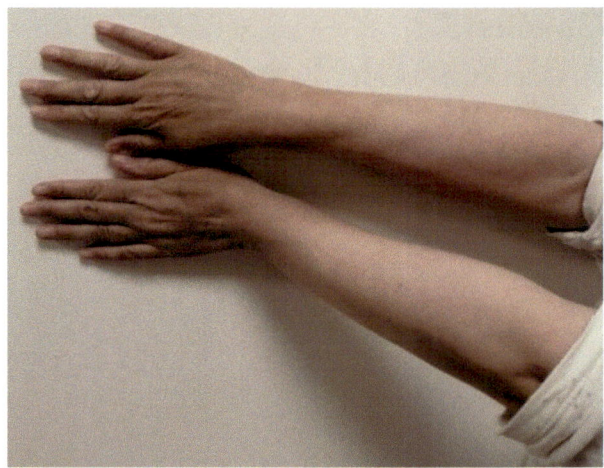

Fig. 3.2 The bilateral
malar fixed erythema and
edema on the eyelids were
presented

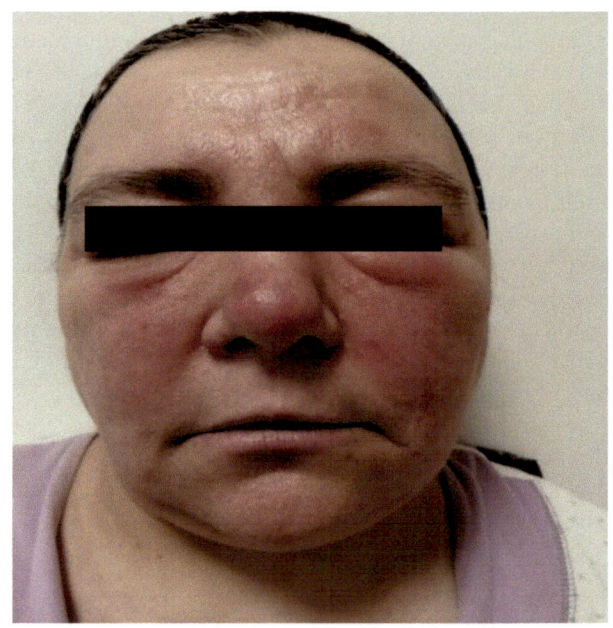

- Peripheral blood smear, posteroanterior (PA) chest X-ray, fecal occult blood test (FOBT), CA 19.9, CA 72.4, CA 125, carcinoembryonic antigen (CEA), alpha-fetoprotein (AFP) and beta-human chorionic gonadotropin (β-HCG) were resulted negative or normal.
- Histopathology: Degeneration of the basal layer and vacuolization, follicular plugging in the epidermis; a mild infiltrate of lymphocyctes in the perivascular and periadnexial area, deposition of dermal mucin in the dermis were observed. Demodex mite was also deteced in the section (Fig. 3.3).

Fig. 3.3 H&E × 40 staining. Histopathology revealed the perifollicular inflammation, lymphocytic infiltration and follicular plugging

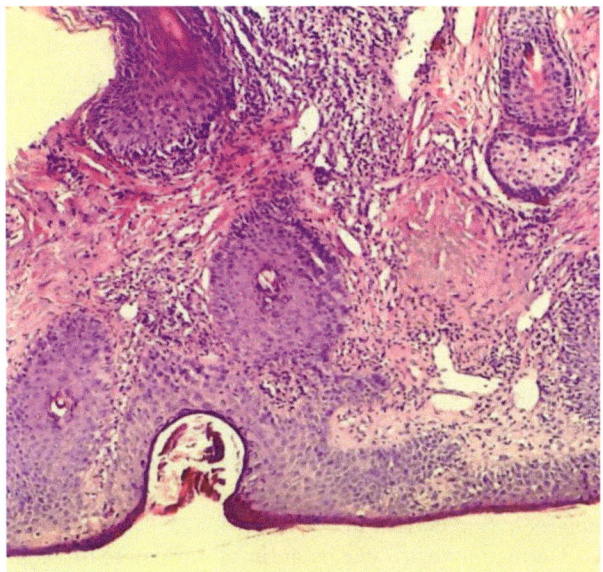

Based on the Description and the Photographs What Is Your Diagnosis?

1. PLE
2. Discoid lupus erythematosus (DLE)
3. Rosacea
4. Dermatomyositis

Diagnosis

DLE.

Discussion

Cutaneous lupus erythematosus (CLE) is a subtype of an autoimmune connective tissue disease that can affect skin, systemic lupus erythematosus (SLE) [1]. DLE, the most common variant of CLE is characterized by dry red or violaceous papules, patches and plaques on the face. It can be presented as papulosquamous or atrophic appearance [2]. Periorbital edema can be a symptom of DLE. A 33-year old woman who developed prominent periorbital edema and erythema diagnosed as DLE was reported [3]. Although the exact role of demodex mites in DLE etiopathogenesis is not known, the presence of high demodex density in DLE patients has been reported [4]. In this case, the patient has Demodex positive-DLE consistent with clinical and histopathological evaluation.

In differential diagnosis, PLE, the most common type of idiopathic photodermatosis is a recurrent, delayed rash caused by sunlight that occurs in susceptible individuals after exposure to ultraviolet (UV) radiation. It starts during the second or third decades of life and commonly affects outdoors workers. Classical papulovesicular lesions are usually disturbed symmetrically on some sun-exposed areas of the skin such as the arms and V-area of the chest [5]. In the absence of this clinical appearance and chronic UV exposure history, we excluded PLE.

Although the patient had a rash compatible with the erythematotelangiectatic type rosacea in the form of bilateral fixed erythema in the malar areas on the face, rosacea was excluded due to the absence of rosacea-specific histopathological findings such as extensive telangiectasias throughout the superficial and middle dermis and increased dermal mast cells [6].

Dermatomyositis can be at times difficult to distinguish from DLE in our patient. The periorbital edema was presented. Dermatomyositis was excluded due to the absence of identifiable proximal myopathy (polymyositis), heliotrope rash (violaceous discoloration in the upper eyelids), Gottron's papules (flat-topped, erythematous to violaceous papules on the metacarpophalangeal and interphalangeal joints), periungual telangiectases. Antinuclear antibody test is generally positive in patients with dermatomyositis, unlike our patient [7].

Key Points
- DLE is a chronic inflammatory erythematous skin disease that may be accompanied by demodex mites.
- It is important to consider the history, clinical findings and histopathological evaluation together in the diagnosis of DLE.
- In the presence of chronic erythematous rash and periorbital edema on the face, DLE should also be considered.

References

1. Sota J, Rigante D, Ruscitti P, et al. Anakinra drug retention rate and predictive factors of drug survival in systemic juvenile idiopathic arthritis and adult onset Still's disease. Front Pharmacol. 2019;10:918.
2. Elman SA, Joyce C, Nyberg F, et al. Development of classification criteria for discoid lupus erythematosus: results of a Delphi exercise. J Am Acad Dermatol. 2017;77(2):261–7.
3. Serarslan G, Atik E, Sarikaya G. Periorbital edema and erythema: an unusual localization of DLE in a patient with psoriasis. J Dermatol. 2011;38(5):486–8.

4. Dursun R, Durmaz K, Oltulu P, Ataseven A. Demodex positive discoid lupus erythematosus: is it a separate entity or an overlap syndrome? Dermatol Ther. 2020:e13394.
5. Hönigsmann H. Polymorphous light eruption. Photodermatol Photoimmunol Photomed. 2008;24(3):155–61.
6. Cribier B. Rosacea under the microscope: characteristic histological findings. J Eur Acad Dermatol Venereol. 2013;27(11):1336–43.
7. Callen JP. Dermatomyositis. Lancet. 2000;355(9197):53–7.

Chapter 4
A Case of Stubborn Facial Redness

Sabha Mushtaq

Case Presentation

A 51 year old female presented to the Dermatology outpatient clinic with chief complains of burning and redness over the face since 5 months. Her symptoms used to aggravate on exposure to sunlight and heat. She had been applying over the counter topical corticosteroids (Betamethasone valerate and clobetasol propionate) on her face as a daily cream for about an year. The patient started using topical corticosteroids as fairness cream and subsequently to relieve the itching and redness which used to occur on their cessation. Patient reported that the redness was transient to begin with but since 5 months it had been persistent, not relieved by application of topical steroids. The obstinate facial redness was a source of cosmetic disfigurement for the patient and had significantly affected her social life. There was no history of fever, joint pains, oral ulcers, ocular complains or Raynaud's phenomenon. The patient was otherwise healthy with no systemic complains.

General physical examination and laboratory parameters were within normal limits. Cutaneous examination revealed erythema over the face predominantly involving the cheeks and sparing the nasolabial folds. On closer examination, numerous linear and arborizing telangiectases were noted over the cheeks on a background of pinkish erythema (Fig. 4.1). The skin over the cheeks was thinned out and atrophic. Oral and ocular examination did not reveal any abnormality.

S. Mushtaq (✉)
Department of Dermatology, Venereology & Leprology, Government Medical College and Associated Hospitals, Jammu, University of Jammu, Jammu and Kashmir, India

© The Author(s), under exclusive license to Springer Nature Switzerland AG 2022
T. M. Lotti et al. (eds.), *Clinical Cases in Facial Erythema*, Clinical Cases in Dermatology, https://doi.org/10.1007/978-3-031-05996-4_4

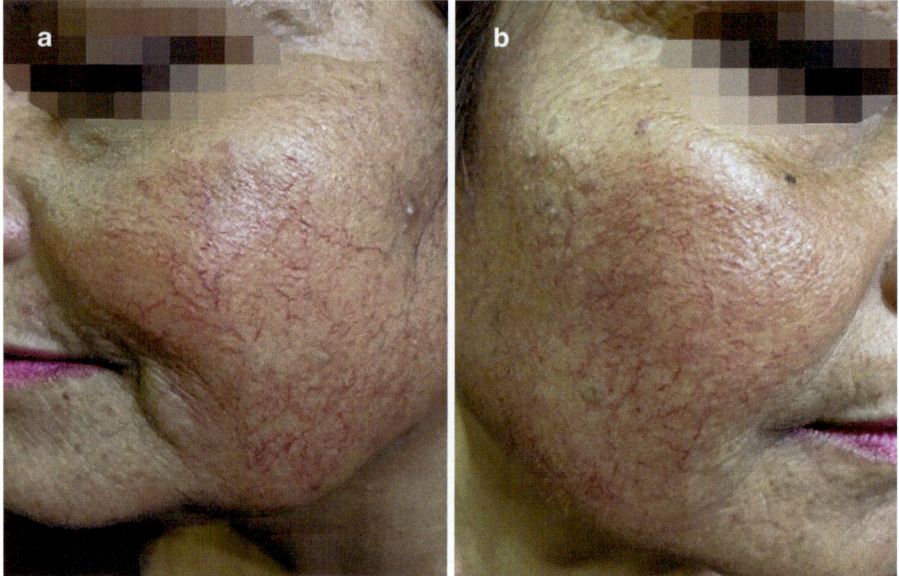

Fig. 4.1 (**a**, **b**) Linear and arborizing telangiectases on a background of pinkish erythema over bilateral cheeks

What Is Your Diagnosis?

- Rosacea
- Lupus erythematosus (LE)
- Scleroderma

Diagnosis

Topical steroid damaged/dependent face (TSDF).

Discussion

Misuse of topical corticosteroids (TCS) on the face was first reported from India in 2006 in a series of five cases that developed facial dermatitis similar to rosacea on prolonged use of TCS creams as cosmetic creams [1]. The condition has been reported under various names in literature such as red skin syndrome, steroid-induced rosacea like dermatitis and dermatitis rosaceiformis steroidica [2, 3]. Topical steroid damaged/dependent face (TSDF) is damage to the facial skin caused by unsupervised, prolonged and indiscriminate use of TCS. It can present as a variety of signs and symptoms like atrophy, striae, dryness, erythema, acneiform eruption, perioral dermatitis, pigmentary changes, telangiectases, rosacea-like picture and allergic contact dermatitis. Besides the clinical damage to the facial skin, patient develops psychological dependence on TCS leading to the latter being abused and misused [2, 4]. Diagnosis of the condition is clinched from a detailed history which would reveal that the TCS were started for a primary facial dermatosis like melasma and acne followed by their continued use in an attempt to relieve the withdrawal effects caused by their abrupt stoppage. The severity of damage depends on various factors such as the age group, site of abuse and potency of TCS used. Facial skin is thinner than other body areas making it more vulnerable to TCS induced damage [2]. Treatment involves withdrawal of the TCS, emollients, topical tacrolimus and antihistamines. Other drugs which have been tried include doxycycline, minocycline and metronidazole. Psychological support and counselling form a crucial part of management besides the medical treatment, to break the vicious cycle [2, 4].

Rosacea is a chronic inflammatory skin condition with a remitting and relapsing course and mostly occurring in people with fair complexion. Convexities of the central face are typically involved. The primary features include flushing, erythema, telangiectases, papules and pustules. Burning/stinging, edema, phymatous changes and ocular involvement are secondary features which may accompany the primary signs and symptoms or occur independently in some cases [5]. Cutaneous atrophy is not a feature of rosacea.

Lupus erythematosus (LE) is an autoimmune connective tissue disorder that affects the skin and other organ systems. The mucocutaneous manifestations of LE include malar rash, discoid rash, photosensitivity, lupus hair and oral/nasal ulcers. The clinical presentation varies as per the disease subtypes. Malar rash or butterfly rash is a flat or raised erythematous rash, characteristic of acute cutaneous LE. It typically involves the butterfly distribution of the face i.e. across the cheeks and bridge of nose, sparing the nasolabial folds. Photosensitivity is usually present with history of appearance of rash or its exacerbation after sun exposure, lasting from days to weeks. Pain and pruritus are occasionally reported with the rash [6].

Scleroderma is a chronic connective tissue disease characterised by Raynaud's phenomenon and skin sclerosis along with systemic symptoms related to internal organ involvement. Limited scleroderma also called as CREST syndrome shows Raynaud's phenomenon and skin sclerosis limited to the face and extremities distal to the elbows and knees. Facial erythema is usually not a feature of scleroderma but telangiectases are commonly observed, more frequently in limited scleroderma than diffuse. Telangiectases can be be mat like or stellate and are primarily seen on the face, hands and fingers [7].

Key Points
- Psychological and physical dependence on TCS leads to their misuse which has deleterious effects on the skin.
- Facial skin is particularly susceptible to the harmful effects of TCS which presents as a range of features like xerosis, itching, erythema, telangiectases and perioral dermatitis. This phenomenon has been described as TSDF.

- TSDF is a source of cosmetic disfigurement to the patient.
- Failure to recognise this clinical entity at an early stage can result in irreversible skin damage.
- Withdrawal of TCS along with counselling the patient regarding the side effects of prolonged and inappropriate use of TCS is the mainstay of treatment.

References

1. Rathi S. Abuse of topical steroid as cosmetic cream: a social background of steroid dermatitis. Indian J Dermatol. 2006;51:154–5.
2. Verma S, Madhu R. The great Indian epidemic of superficial dermatophytosis: an appraisal. Indian J Dermatol. 2017;62:227.
3. Rapaport MJ, Rapaport V. The red skin syndromes: corticosteroid addiction and withdrawal. Expert Rev Dermatol. 2006;1:547–61.
4. Saraswat A, Lahiri K, Chatterjee M, Barua S, Coondoo A, Mittal A, Panda S, Rajagopalan M, Sharma R, Abraham A, Verma SB. Topical corticosteroid abuse on the face: a prospective, multicenter study of dermatology outpatients. Indian J Dermatol, Venereol, and Leprol. 2011;77:160.
5. Mikkelsen CS, Holmgren HR, Kjellman P, Heidenheim M, Kappinnen A, Bjerring P, Huldt-Nystrøm T. Rosacea: a clinical review. Dermatol Rep. 2016;15:8.
6. Uva L, Miguel D, Pinheiro C, Freitas JP, Marques Gomes M, Filipe P. Cutaneous manifestations of systemic lupus erythematosus. Autoimmune Dis. 2012;2012
7. Sobolewski P, Maślińska M, Wieczorek M, Łagun Z, Malewska A, Roszkiewicz M, Nitskovich R, Szymańska E, Walecka I. Systemic sclerosis–multidisciplinary disease: clinical features and treatment. Reumatologia. 2019;57:221.

Chapter 5
A Female in Middle Age with Red Nodule

Runping Fang, Lu Wang, Rongming Yang, Shuanglin Li, and Yuan Li

The patient, 48 years old, was presented with a red nodule on her left maxillofacial region. The red nodule has grown bigger in the past 2 months (Fig. 5.1), with purulent secretions discharged intermittently but no pruritus or pain, still not recovered.

Based on the Case Description and the Photograph, What Is Your Diagnosis?

1. Keratoacanthoma
2. Sporotrichosis
3. Dental Sinus
4. Dermatofibrosarcoma Protuberans
5. Pyogenic Granuloma

R. Fang (✉)
Department of Dermatology, Shangyou County People's Hospital, Jiangxi Province, Ganzhou, China

L. Wang
Department of Dermatology, Sichuan Women's and Children's Hospital, Chengdu, Sichuan, China

R. Yang
Department of Dermatology, Shangyou People's Hospital, Ganzhou, China

S. Li
Department of Dermatology, Juxian Hospital of Traditional Chinese Medicine, Rizhao, Shandong, China

Y. Li
Department of Dermatology, Tangshan Huatuo's Hospital, Tangshan, Hebei, China

© The Author(s), under exclusive license to Springer Nature Switzerland AG 2022
T. M. Lotti et al. (eds.), *Clinical Cases in Facial Erythema*, Clinical Cases in Dermatology, https://doi.org/10.1007/978-3-031-05996-4_5

19

Fig. 5.1 Red nodules on
her left maxillofacial
region

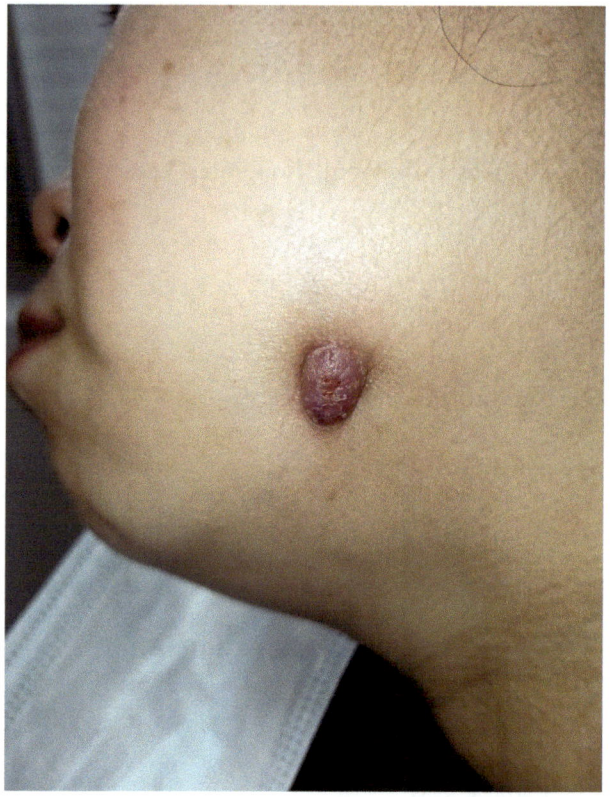

For a long time, she has suffered from toothache. Physical examination showed that
all her molars on the left side of the bottom were decayed, with inflammation around
the root, especially the third molar (Fig. 5.2). In the mandibular angle skin of it
appeared a nodule, which is about 0.8 × 0.6 cm in size, with sunken skin around it.
No other nodules were observed. No systematical treatment was taken for her dental
caries. Once had skin nodules applied medication on her own, but with no effect.

CT examination revealed that a tubular soft tissue density was found under the
skin of the left mandible, leading to the bone area of the mandible and the subcutaneous elliptical low-density shadow of the lateral assessor muscle, CT value is from
35 to 60HU (Fig. 5.3).

Diagnosis

Dental Sinus.

Fig. 5.2 Decayed molars on the left side of the bottom, with inflammation around the root

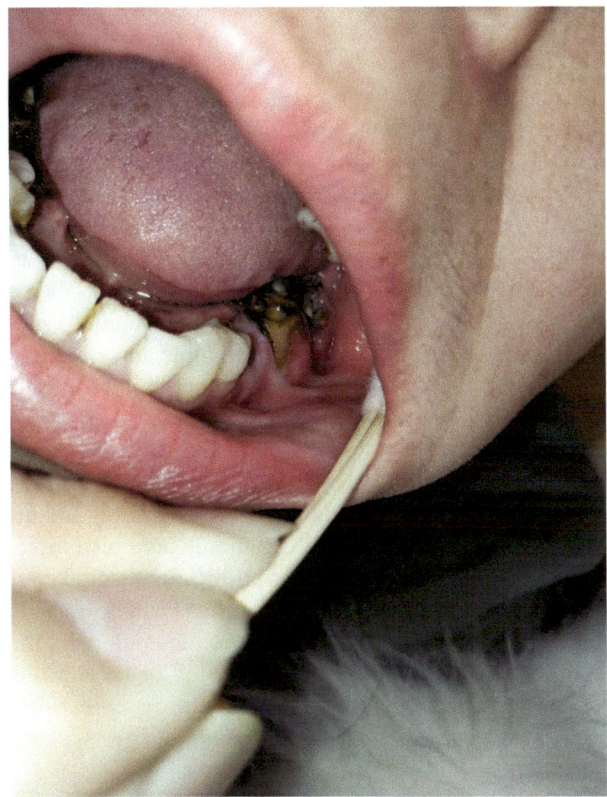

Fig. 5.3 CT scan showed a fistula between the skin and bone in the left mandible

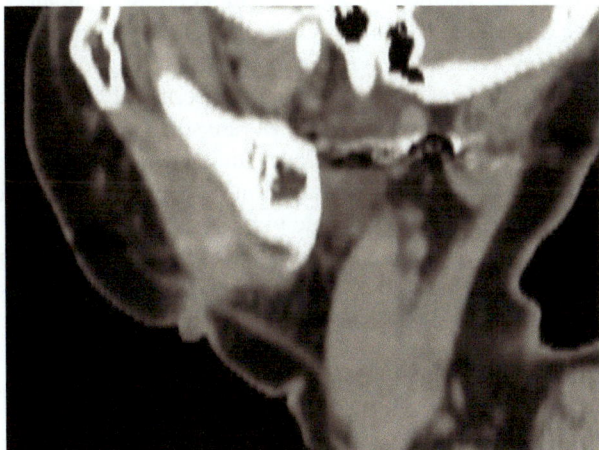

Discussion

Dental Sinus is caused by chronic infection around the root tip of teeth, especially the asymptomatic sinus tract that eventually appears in the gingival, palatal or perioral skin and forms fistulas. The cutaneous opening of the fistula is a small inflammatory red nodule, which could occur anywhere from the inner canthus to the neck, but is most common in the chin or along the jaw line [1].

Odontogenic Cutaneous Sinus Tract is a pathologic canal occurs in the oral cavity and exposes on the cutaneous surface of one's face or neck. Frequent misdiagnosis leads to its inaccurate treatment, but once it diagnosed correctly, oral therapy to eliminate the infective source is a simple and effective treatment [2].

Keratoacanthoma (KA) is a low-grade, rapidly growing, 1–2 cm dome-shaped skin tumor with a centralized keratinous plug. Initial rapid growth, following a period of variable tumor stability, then finally spontaneous regression are characteristics of it. Although recognized as benign, KA shares histopathological features with squamous cell carcinoma (SCC) requiring treatment. It is a highly differentiated form of squamous cell carcinoma, and histological examination reveals a circumscribed proliferation of well-differentiated keratinocytes, which is different from nodules of Dental Sinus. KA has been described as multilobular exophytic or endophytic cyst-like invagination of the epidermis, the epidermis extends over the tumor, and there is a central horn plug of keratin. Peripheral to the keratin-filled crater are lip-like peripheral borders of the epidermis. Intraepidermal neutrophilic abscesses are visualized in addition to horn pearls. The cells of the keratoacanthoma are enlarged and atypical keratinocytes [3].

Sporotrichosis is worth mentioning in the differential diagnosis of this patient. It shares similar clinical features of Dental Sinus. Sporotrichosis is classified into cutaneous, pulmonary, and disseminated, with cutaneous the most common form of the disease. The skin form presents as papules or pustules that form ulcerated nodules involving local lymphatics. Definite diagnosis depends on fungal culture [4].

The clinical manifestations of Dermatofibrosarcoma Protuberans (DFSP) are like those of dental sinus. It is a rare soft tissue tumor that involves the dermis, subcutaneous fat, and in rare cases, muscle and fascia. The tumor typically presents as a slowly growing, firm plaque on the trunk of young adults. The cause of DFSP is not clear. Diagnosis is made via skin biopsy [5].

Pyogenic Granuloma is a common, acquired, benign, vascular tumor which is easily confused with the red nodule of dental sinus. It shows rapid exophytic growth, with a surface that often undergoes ulceration.

Based on the patient's medical history, clinical picture, and imagological examination results, the diagnosis is Dental Sinus. Of note, the use of contrast media can accurately show the shape of fistula.

Surgery is the first choice for the treatment of Dental Sinus. The specific method is to completely remove the fistula and properly close the fistula at both ends, and at the same time eradicate the dental disease.

Key Points
- Dental sinus is a kind of skin lesion caused by odontopathy. Its essence is pathological sinus.
- Lesion most located in the chin or along the jaw line distribution

References

1. Zhao B. Chinese clinical dermatology [M]. Nanjing: Jiangsu Science and Technology Press; 2010. p. 1323–4.
2. Al-Obaida MI, Al-Madi EM. Cutaneous draining sinus tract of odontogenic origin. A case of chronic misdiagnosis. Saudi Med J. 2019;40(3):292–7. https://doi.org/10.15537/smj.2019.3.23963.
3. Zito PM, Scharf R. Keratoacanthoma. 2020 Sep 29. In: StatPearls [Internet]. Treasure Island (FL): StatPearls Publishing; 2020.
4. Sizar O, Talati R. Sporotrichosis. 2020 Jun 30. In: StatPearls [Internet]. Treasure Island (FL): StatPearls Publishing; 2020.
5. Brooks J, Ramsey ML. Dermatofibrosarcoma Protuberans. 2020 Nov 17. In: StatPearls [Internet]. Treasure Island (FL): StatPearls Publishing; 2020.

Chapter 6
A Female with Erythema and Telangiectasis

Ling Yu, Jian-Bo Wang, Shu-Zhen Zhang, and Shou-Min Zhang

A 56-year-old female presented to our clinic complaining of the erythema and telangiectasis on her face back-and-forth 9 months (Fig. 6.1), which aggravated lately and spread to the trunk. There were no any pain, pruritus or any other discomfort symptoms.

Based on the Case Description and Photograph, What Is your Diagnosis?

1. contact dermatitis
2. discoid lupus erythematosus
3. Jessner lymphocytic infiltration of the skin
4. sarcoidosis

Skin biopsies showed multiple non-caseous necrotic epithelium granulomas composed of histiocytes surrounded by a rim of lymphocytes consistent with the diagnosis of sarcoidosis. Then Chest computed tomography was examined and showed multiple lymph nodes enlargement in the mediastinum and pulmonary micro-nodules. Bronchoscopy and biopsy of pulmonary nodule were performed and the result showed granulomatous change also consistent with sarcoidosis, meanwhile, Acid-fast staining and TB-DNA were negative, which excluded tuberculosis. In addition, immunohistochemical staining results excluded the potential malignancy.

L. Yu · J.-B. Wang · S.-Z. Zhang · S.-M. Zhang (✉)
Department of Dermatology, Henan Provincial People's Hospital, People's Hospital of Zhengzhou University, People's Hospital of Henan University, Zhengzhou, China

© The Author(s), under exclusive license to Springer Nature
Switzerland AG 2022
T. M. Lotti et al. (eds.), *Clinical Cases in Facial Erythema*, Clinical Cases in
Dermatology, https://doi.org/10.1007/978-3-031-05996-4_6

Fig. 6.1 The erythema and
telangiectasis on her face

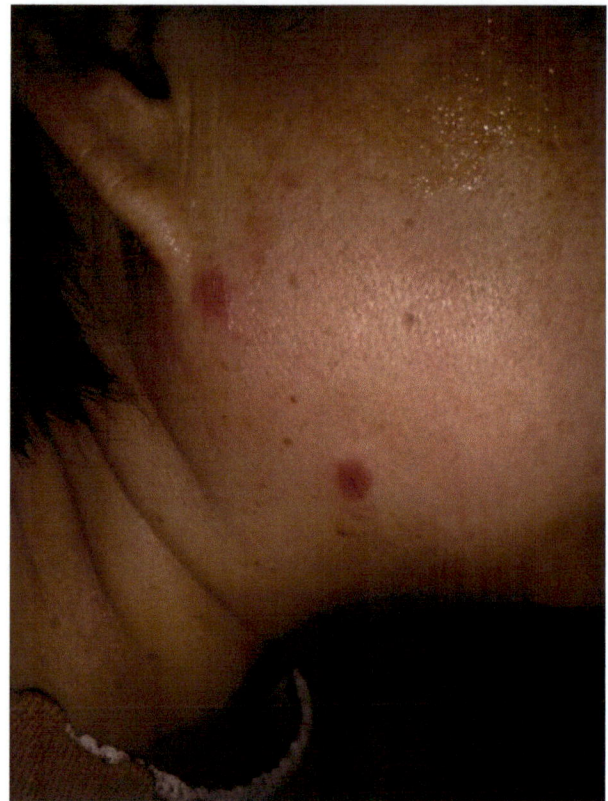

Diagnosis

Sarcoidosis.

Discussion

Sarcoidosis is a kind of chronic multisystemic inflammatory disease defined by the
presence of non-caseating granulomas with unknown etiology. It can affect a number of organs, most commonly the lungs, lymph nodes and skin. Cutaneous lesions
may have a variety of presentations including papules, plaques, nodules, infiltrative
scars, annular, angiolupoid, psoriasiform, hypopigmented, atrophic, ulcerative
lesions, scarring and nonscarring alopecia, erythroderma, and ichthyosiform lesions
[1]. Since it can mimic many other cutaneous diseases, it also earning the term of"a
great imitator".

Contact dermatitis is acute or chronic inflammatory cutaneous disease that is caused by substances contacted with the skin. We can find the precipitating factors in contact dermatitis patients, whose lesions are always confined to areas exposed to offending agents.

Discoid lupus erythematosus is an autoimmune disease charcaterized by manifestations of erythema, scaling, atrophy, dyspigmentation, scarring and alopecia. The lesions are found most often on the face, scalp and ears, which can be exacerbated once exposing to the sun. Histology shows focal interface dermatitis and dense perivascular and periadnexal lymphoid infiltrates throughout the entire dermis [2]. The histopathological examination can help differentiate sarcoidsis easily.

Jessner lymphocytic infiltration of the skin is a rare, benign cutaneous condition characterized by non-scaly erythema, papular or plaque-like eruptions that commonly involve sun-exposed areas such as face, neck, and trunk. This disease has an indolent course. The eruptions may clear spontaneously or with the aid of medications. The lesions are usually asymptomatic, but frequently recur. It is diagnosed by biopsy revealing perivascular and periadnexal clusters of plasmacytoid monocytes within the dermis, sometimes extending into the subcutaneous tissue [3].

Based on the patient's clinical manifestation, chest CT imaging findings and biopsy results of skin and lung nodule, the diagnosis of sarcoidosis was made. The lesions on this patient manifest like angiolupoid, which is also one of uncommon presentations of sarcoidosis. The accepted first-line therapy for cutaneous sarcoidosis consists of intralesional and oral corticosteroids, so oral prednisone was prescribed and the lesions and lung nodules were gradually relief.

Key Points
- Sarcoidosis is a chronic multisystemic inflammatory disease defined by the presence of non-caseating granulomas with unknown etiology. It can affect a number of organs, most commonly the lungs, lymph nodes and skin.
- It is a great imitator, the cutaneous lesions may have a variety of presentations.

References

1. Karadağ P, et al. Sarcoidosis: A great imitator. Clin Dermatol. 2019;37(3):240–54.
2. Bolognia S, et al. Dermatology. 3th ed. Elsevier; 2012.
3. Williams H, et al. Jessner lymphocytic infiltration of the skin. Treasure Island (FL); 2020.

Chapter 7
A Female with Nodules

Yining Wang and Xing-Hua Gao

A 61-year-old female presented to the clinic complaining of painless erythematous nodules on the face and back that had occurred for a year.

Based on the case description and the photograph, what is your diagnosis?

1. Cutaneous Rosai-Dorfman Disease
2. Langerhan cell histiocytosis (LCH)
3. juvenile xanthogranuloma (JXG)
4. IgG4-related disease

One year ago, a 5 mm red papule occurred on the back, followed by another 1 cm red papule on the nose 4 months later (Fig. 7.1). The first biopsy was taken from back skin for pathological test, while diagnosis was undetermined. Treatment with 0.03% tacrolimus ointment for half a month had no effect. Another biopsy was taken from back skin again for the second pathological test. The pathological diagnosis was cutaneous Rosai-Dorfman disease. Treatment with fluticasone propionate cream and ketoprofen gel four to five times per day for one month showed no effect. Then, compound betamethasone (betamethasone dipropionate (calculated as betamethasone) 5 mg and betamethasone sodium phosphate (calculated as betamethasone) 2 mg) intralesional injection was additionally given twice, combined with use of 0.1% tacrolimus ointment. No effective outcome occurred. Bleomycin hydrochloride intralesional injection once showed no effect either.

H&E staining showed focal inflammatory cells aggregation in the dermis and subcutaneous tissue. Intact lymphocytes and plasma cells were seen in the abundant pale cytoplasm of the enlarged histiocytes (emperipolesis). Histiocytes were positive for CD68, CD163 and S100, and negative for CD38 and CD1a.

Y. Wang · X.-H. Gao (✉)
Department of Dermatology, The First Hospital of China Medical University,
Shenyang, China

© The Author(s), under exclusive license to Springer Nature
Switzerland AG 2022
T. M. Lotti et al. (eds.), *Clinical Cases in Facial Erythema*, Clinical Cases in
Dermatology, https://doi.org/10.1007/978-3-031-05996-4_7

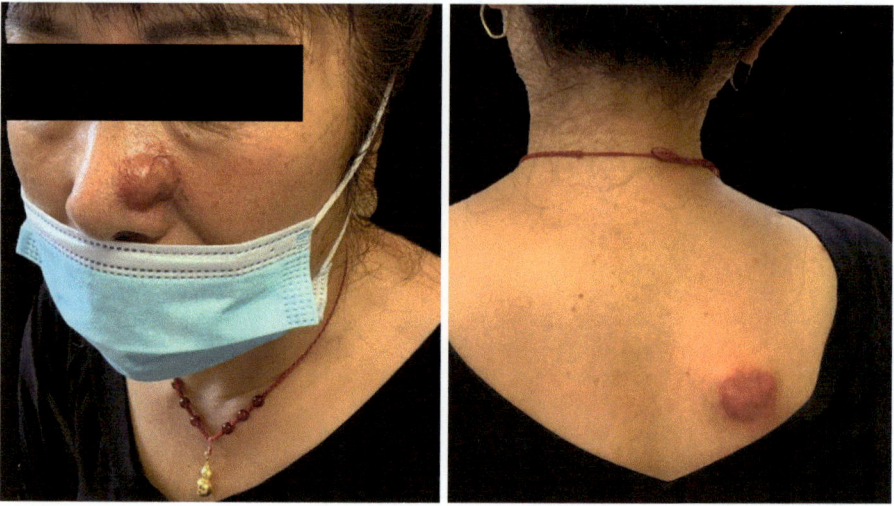

Fig. 7.1 A 61-year-old female presented to the clinic complaining of painless erythematous nodule on the face and back that had occurred for a year

Diagnosis

Cutaneous Rosai-Dorfman Disease.

Discussion

Rosai-Dorfman-Destombes disease (RDD) is a rare histiocytic disorder described as 'sinus histiocytosis with massive lymphadenopathy (SHML)'. Kinase mutations have been described in nodal and extranodal (but not cutaneous) RDD, including mutations in *ARAF*, *MAP 2 K1*, *NRAS* and *KRAS*. *BRAF V600E* mutations have also been sought in RDD. No data on the molecular profile of cutaneous RDD could be found [1].

Cutaneous RDD demonstrates unique epidemiological and clinical features. Cutaneous RDD presents in patients with an older mean age (43.5 years) than nodal RDD (20.6 years), a higher proportion of female patients (2:1 ratio) and a higher proportion of Asian and white patients. The most common clinical presentation was that of slowly growing cutaneous nodules or papules ranging from less than 1 cm to 9 cm in maximum dimension [2]. Other presentations described include indurated plaques, tumour-like lesions, acne-form lesions and eruptive xanthoma-like lesions. The lesions were distributed over the trunk, face, and extremities, and can be solitary, clustering or multiple affecting different anatomical sites. Cutaneous RDD patients typically lack an association with visceral organ involvement or lymphadenopathy, and the disease process tends to remain localized despite long-term follow-up [1–3]. Surgical excision may be indicated in unifocal extranodal disease or for symptomatic airway, cranial, spinal or sinus disease. Those with multifocal irresectable extranodal disease may require systemic therapy of which there is currently no standardised regimen. Systemic therapies include corticosteroids, sirolimus, radiotherapy, chemotherapy and immunomodulatory therapy [4]. High dose thalidomide, vincristine, methotrexate, acitretin, isoretinoid and dapsone have been used with measurable success for aggressive and refractory disease. Steroids have shown to be least effective with several cases undergoing remission after stopping its use [5].

The most important differential diagnosis of RDD is that of Langerhans cell histiocytosis (LCH). LCH is an inflammatory myeloid neoplasm of mixed cellularity. A diagnosis of RDD by definition requires the exclusion of LCH by negative CD1a or CD207 staining of the histiocytic infiltrate. Other morphological clues to this differential are the absence of an eosinophilic infiltrate in RDD, the characteristic elongated grooved nuclear features of LCH and the absence of a prominent plasma cell component in LCH. Of note, S100 positivity is observed in both RDD and LCH. RDD may be associated with LCH [1].

Cutaneous RDD must be distinguished from juvenile xanthogranuloma (JXG). JXG is a benign, self-healing disorder characterized by solitary or multiple yellow-red nodules. It is predominantly a disease of infancy or early childhood. Histologically, JXG represents an accumulation of histiocytes lacking Birbeck granules (non-Langerhans cells). JXG is characterized by the presence of Touton cells showing the typical "wreath" of nuclei surrounded by foamy cytoplasm, negativity for S100 and lack of emperipolesis [1].

RDD may share some morphological features with IgG4-related disease, such as storiform fibrosis and abundant plasma cells. The main distinguishing feature supportive of cutaneous RDD would be the extent of histiocytic infiltration, the presence of emperilopolesis and the classic phenotypic profile. In 2015, an expert panel stated neither clinical or pathological features alone are sufficient to make a diagnosis of IgG4-related disease and that disorders that mimic IgG4-related disease must be rigorously excluded [6]. All cases of RDD should be evaluated for IgG4-positive plasma cell infiltration (based on expert opinion: grade D2 evidence) [7].

Based on the patient's medical history, clinical pictures and biopsy results, the diagnosis of cutaneous Rosai-Dorfman disease was made. The large histiocytes with abundant pale cytoplasm and the identification of emperipolesis are characteristic. The histiocytes are S100, CD68 and CD163 positive and are CD1a negative, thereby excluding LCH. CD38 negativity demonstrated no abundant plasma cells, which was insufficient for IgG4-related disease diagnosis.

Oral thalidomide was prescribed at a dose of 100 mg per day. The nodule became thinner with lightened redness and slight scale after 2 months. Facial redness and swelling led to the discontinuation of the medication and administration of thalidomide restarted after the symptoms disappeared in a month. During the medication, new red papules occurred on the cheek and scapular area. The nodule on the nose became slightly bigger and more firm.

Key Points
- Cutaneous Rosai-Dorfman Disease is persistent, benign and can be associated with involvement of other organs or with immune mediated diseases.
- The S100-positive histiocytes with emperipolesis that impart a dark and light zonal appearance to the tissue are characteristic. Immunohistochemistry and close attention to the H&E morphology can resolve most of the differentials.

References

1. Bruce-Brand C, Schneider JW, Schubert P. Rosai-Dorfman disease: an overview. J Clin Pathol. 2020;73(11):697–705.
2. Brenn T, Calonje E, Granter SR, Leonard N, Grayson W, Fletcher CDM, et al. Cutaneous rosai-dorfman disease is a distinct clinical entity. Am J Dermatopathol. 2002;24(5):385–91.
3. Kong Y-Y, Kong J-C, Shi D-R, Lu H-F, Zhu X-Z, Wang J, et al. Cutaneous rosai-dorfman disease: a clinical and histopathologic study of 25 cases in China. Am J Surg Pathol. 2007;31(3):341–50.
4. Abla O, Jacobsen E, Picarsic J, Krenova Z, Jaffe R, Emile J-F, et al. Consensus recommendations for the diagnosis and clinical management of Rosai-Dorfman-Destombes disease. Blood. 2018;131(26):2877–90.
5. Ahmed A, Crowson N, Magro CM. A comprehensive assessment of cutaneous Rosai-Dorfman disease. Ann Diagn Pathol. 2019;40:166–73.
6. Khosroshahi A, Wallace ZS, Crowe JL, Akamizu T, Azumi A, Carruthers MN, et al. International consensus guidance statement on the management and treatment of IgG4-related disease. Arthritis Rheumatol. 2015;67(7):1688–99.
7. Emile J-F, Abla O, Fraitag S, Horne A, Haroche J, Donadieu J, et al. Revised classification of histiocytoses and neoplasms of the macrophage-dendritic cell lineages. Blood. 2016;127(22):2672–81.

Chapter 8
A Female with Thick Crust on Lip

Jing Lan, Wei Huo, Hao Guo, Qian An, and Xing-Hua Gao

A 60-year old lady presented to the office with her son complaining of thick, swollen and crusted lesion on her lip with occasional pain that has lasted for 1 year long (Fig. 8.1).

Baed on the case description and the photograph, what is your diagnosis?

1. Cheilitis
2. Psoriasis
3. Lichen planus
4. Lupus erythematosus
5. Contact dermatitis

She had used several kinds of glucocorticoids ointment irregularly that partially controlled the symptoms; while stopping the drugs results in flaring up. She also used ketoconazole ointment a couple of days, but to no avail. Her general health was

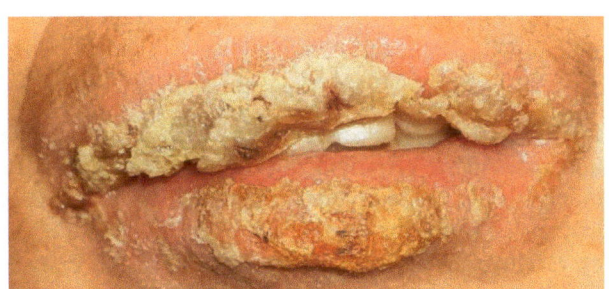

Fig. 8.1 Clinical manifestation of the patient. Diffuse erythematous swelling and slight exudation of her lips, covered by thick, dry, and yellowish crust

J. Lan · W. Huo · H. Guo · Q. An · X.-H. Gao (✉)
Department of Dermatology, The First Hospital of China Medical University,
Shenyang, China

© The Author(s), under exclusive license to Springer Nature
Switzerland AG 2022
T. M. Lotti et al. (eds.), *Clinical Cases in Facial Erythema*, Clinical Cases in
Dermatology, https://doi.org/10.1007/978-3-031-05996-4_8

Fig. 8.2 Biopsy specimen revealed that superficial perivascular lymphocytic infiltrate with overlying epidermal acanthosis; prominent spongiosis with exocytosis of lymphocytes compatible with spongiotic dermatitis (HEx20)

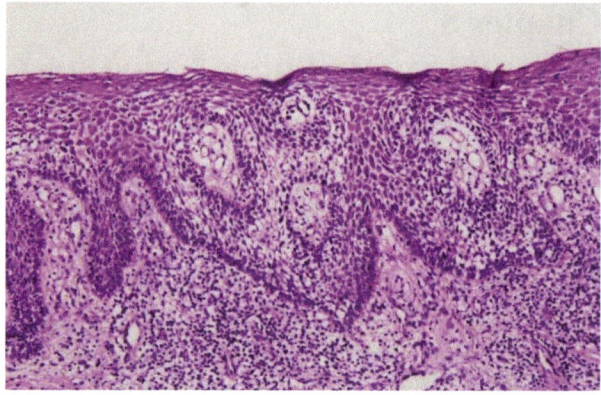

good. On presentation, there was diffuse erythematous swelling and slight exudation of her lips, covered by thick, dry, and yellowish crust (Fig. 8.1). Her oral mucosa and other parts of the skin were intact.

The biopsy specimen taken from the lower lip revealed a superficial perivascular lymphocytic infiltrate with overlying epidermal acanthosis; promiment spongiosis with exocytosis of lymphocytes compatible with spongiotic dermatitis (Fig. 8.2). Fungi identification by microscopy was negative. Patch test for the topical creams she had used to apply was negative.

Diagnosis

Crusted Cheilitis.

Discussion

Cheilitis is an inflammation of lip, which could be acute or chronic. The inflammation arises in the vermilion zone but may extend to surrounding skin and less commonly, to the oral mucosa. It may be caused by lots of factors, including contact irritants or allergens, chronic sun exposure, and nutritional deficiencies, as well as by various cutaneous and systemic diseases [1]. Exogenous factors (irritant contact cheilitis and allergic cheilitis), endogenous factors and frequent exposure to hot or dry winds are the most common causes; besides, a variety of other substances that come into contact with lips also increase the incidence of the disease [2]. Patients with a history of atopy or atopic dermatitis usually present with dryness, erythema, scaling and fissuring on lips [3]. Some cheilitis are even caused by infections such as virus (especially type 1 herpes simplex virus), bacteria (group A Streptococcus or Staphylococcus) [4] or fungi [5]. Furthermore, cheilitis can also be seen in various

Fig. 8.3 Crust was removed after one-month treatment with topical compound flumetasone and salicylic acid ointment

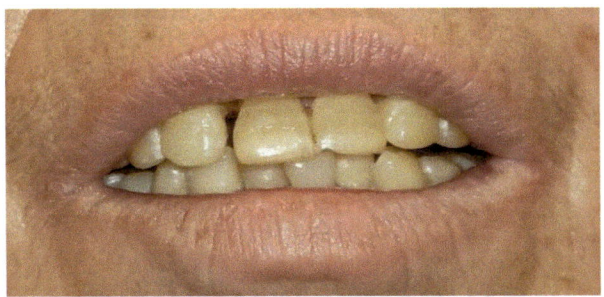

skin or systemic diseases such as lupus erythematosus, lichen planus, atopic dermatitis, megaloblastic anemia due to vitamin B12 deficiency, anemia due to iron deficiency and diabetes. In the present case, the patient had gotten neither the history of atopy or atopic dermatitis nor positive results of patch test applied on her skin, suggesting that her lip inflammation was probably not induced by contact substance. In addition, her physical condition is good. In order to further exclude autoimmune disease, we took specimen from her lower lip and pathological exam showed superficial perivascular lymphocytic infiltrate with overlying epidermal acanthosis and promiment spongiosis with exocytosis of lymphocytes compatible with spongiotic dermatitis, indicating a typical characteristic of cheilitis. According to theses inspection items, we speculated that the cheilitis may due to dehydration induced by bad habits like frequently licking or scratching.

Management for cheilitis firstly depends on avoiding etiological factors. For physical stimulation induced dry, chapped lips, avoidance of lip sucking, lip balms and the local application of petroleum jelly is helpful [6]. Topical antiseptics/antibiotics or fungicidal medications are applied to inhibit the inflammation induced by infection and oral antibiotics could be used if necessary. Usually topical glucocorticoids could control the disease development if no infection is involved. This patient was instructed to avoid scratching and licking. Meanwhile, topical compound flumetasone and salicylic acid ointment were applied on her lip which well controlled the inflammation after one-month treatment (Fig. 8.3).

Key Points
Cheilitis is inflammation of lips with very complex etiologies which need to be figured out clearly so that the treatment could be worked out accordingly.

References

1. Litaiem N, et al. Cheilitis with hemorrhagic crusts of the vermilion lips. Int J Dermatol. 2020;59(7):e234–6.
2. Griggs J, et al. "fresh breath" on toothpaste: peppermint as cause of Cheilitis. Dermatitis. 2019;30(1):74–5.
3. Farmer WS, et al. Atopic dermatitis: managing the itch. Adv Exp Med Biol. 2017;1027:161–77.

4. Garbacz K, et al. Denture stomatitis associated with small-colony variants of Staphylococcus aureus: a case report. BMC Oral Health. 2019;19(1):219.
5. Baumgardner DJ, et al. Oral fungal microbiota: to thrush and beyond. J Patient Cent Res Rev. 2019;6(4):252–61.
6. Collet E, et al. Cheilitis, perioral dermatitis and contact allergy. Eur J Dermatol. 2013;23(3):303–7.

Chapter 9
A Middle-Aged Male with Multiple Plaques

Xi Wang and Songmei Geng

A 56-year-old Chinese male presents with a six-month history of asymptomatic multiple papules and swelling in face and upper extremities. The lesions were initially dense, waxy, slightly red to flesh colored papules and plaques involving his face, back and limbs, together with a sensation of tightness (Fig. 9.1a). Subsequently, the lesions gradually evolved into widespread infiltrated thickening and sclerosis. Physical exam revealed furrows on the glabella (characteristic Leonine facies) and mild pitting edema (Fig. 9.1b).

Based on the case description and the photograph, what is your diagnosis?

1. systemic sclerosis
2. dermatomyositis
3. lichen myxedematosus
4. chronic graft-versus-host disease

Laboratory findings for complete blood count, urinalysis, liver, and renal function tests were within the normal limits. Test for thyroid function and related tests for connective tissue disease were also normal. Histopathology of skin lesion showed almost normal epidermis and generalized mucin depositing between the irregularly arranged collagen fibers with fibroblast proliferation in dermis. Mildly increased inflammatory cell infiltration was also observed in the dermis (Fig. 9.2a). Special staining with Alcian blue indicated notable mucin deposition (Fig. 9.2b).

X. Wang · S. Geng (✉)
Department of Dermatology, The Second Hospital Affiliated to Xi'an Jiaotong University, Xi'an, China
e-mail: wangxi2016@stu.xjtu.edu.cn

© The Author(s), under exclusive license to Springer Nature Switzerland AG 2022
T. M. Lotti et al. (eds.), *Clinical Cases in Facial Erythema*, Clinical Cases in Dermatology, https://doi.org/10.1007/978-3-031-05996-4_9

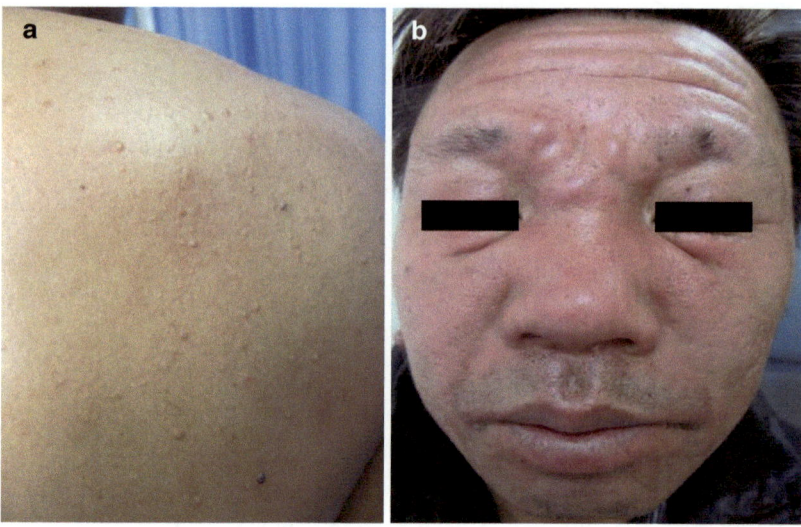

Fig. 9.1 A 56-year-old Chinese male presents with a six-month history of multiple papules and plaques involving his face, back and limb as well as swelling in face and upper extremities. Clinical manifestations of the patient with lichen myxedematosus. (**a**) Multiple papules involving his back and limbs, together with a sensation of tightness; (**b**) Deep furrows were visible on the glabella (characteristic Leonine facies) and mild pitting edema of his face

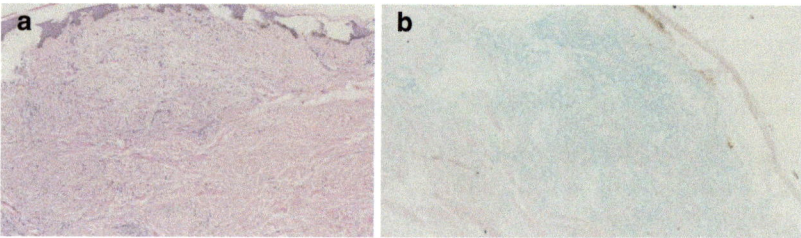

Fig. 9.2 A biopsy was performed at lesions of left forearm. (**a**) hematoxylin and eosin, ×10; (**b**) special staining with Alcian blue, ×10

Diagnosis

lichen myxedematosus.

Discussion

Lichen myxedematosus (LM), an idiopathic cutaneous mucinosis that is not associated with thyroid disease, was first described by Dubreuilh in 1906. Later in 1953, Montgomery and Underwood categorized it into three subsets: (1) generalized LM (scleromyxedema), (2) a localized variant, (3) and an atypical form with features intermediate between the first two [1]. Scleromyxedema is a rare, chronic and unpredictable subtype of the LM family, which may has multiple organs involved and is virtually always in association with monoclonal gammopathy. This disease generally affects middle-aged adults without sex predominance, and usually distributes on the hands and face [2]. Cutaneous manifestations of scleromyxedema are usually generalized, dense, waxy, slightly reddish or skin-colored, dome-shaped or flat papules of 2 to 3 mm diameter, as well as sclerodermoid eruption, which may confers a typical leonine facies or doughnut sign [3]. Histologically, it is characterized by the classic triad of dermal mucin deposition, fibroblast proliferation and fibrosis. However, an interstitial granuloma annulare like pattern was also described in recently published case series [3]. 70% to 77% of patients have been reported suffering from systemic manifestations, including neurologic, hematologic, and cardiologic involvement leading to a guarded prognosis [4]. Nevertheless, due to the unclear pathogenesis of the disease, scleromyxedema currently has no standard treatment, and the therapeutic response varies among different patients [5]. High-dosed intravenous immunoglobulins (IVIg) are considered the first-line treatment according to the guideline [3]. Other treatments that have been frequently used include thalidomide, steroids, autologous stem cell transplantation, and plasma cell-directed therapies.

Systemic sclerosis is a connective tissue disorder characterized by vascular alterations, extensive fibrosis and autoantibodies against various cellular antigens. The lesions are characterized by very densely accumulation of collagen in the dermis, loss of cells, and atrophy. LM may be differentiated from it by Cutaneous findings, which are usually nailfold changes, calcinosis, or telangiectasia in the latter.

Dermatomyositis is a microangiopathy affecting skin and muscle. The typical skin lesions are itching, purple-red papules or plaques, mainly distributing on upper body. Muscular manifestations are usually weakness or inflammation of distal muscles. Muscle weakness can also be observed in LM, while a biopsy will facilely distinguish dermatomyositis from LM which usually shows hyperkeratotic, epidermal atrophy and perivascular lymphocytic infiltrate in the former [6].

Graft-versus-host disease (GVHD) is an immune-mediated syndrome that affects many organ systems. The top ranked target for chronic GVHD is the skin. Cutaneous manifestations are extremely polymorphic, potentially affect all layers of the skin and subcutaneous tissue, and present in the forms of sclerotic and non-sclerotic. Its initial manifestation usually appears within 3 years after allogeneic HCT and are virtually accompanied by a history of acute GVHD.

A diagnosis of lichen myxedematosus was made based on cutaneous findings and histologic observed in the dermis. Most Lab values of our patient were within normal limits. No complications or extracutaneous manifestations were found in this case. We prescribed acitretin, thalidomide and phototherapy to the patient, and the patient's state ameliorated with improvement of skin lesions and disappearance of swelling in his face and upper extremities.

Key Points
- Lichen myxedematosus (LM), an idiopathic cutaneous mucinosis, is characterized by diffuse mucin deposition with fibroblast proliferation in the dermis.
- In this case, differential diagnosis should include systemic sclerosis, dermatomyositis and chronic graft-versus-host disease.
- Currently, the management of scleromyxedema remains a therapeutic challenge. Treatments with acitretin, thalidomide and phototherapy are attended with satisfactory results in this case.

References

1. Vyas NS. Lichen Myxedematosus: case report and review of literature. J Drugs Dermatol. 2020;19(3):320–2.
2. Win H, Gowin K. Treatment of scleromyxedema with lenalidomide, bortezomib and dexamethasone: a case report and review of the literature. Clin Case Rep. 2020;8(12):3043–9.
3. Hoffmann JHO, Enk AH. Scleromyxedema. J Dtsch Dermatol Ges. 2020;18(12):1449–67.
4. Cárdenas-Gonzalez RE, Ruelas MEH, Candiani JO. Lichen myxedematosus: a rare group of cutaneous mucinosis. An Bras Dermatol. 2019;94(4):462–9.
5. Rongioletti F, Merlo G, Cinotti E, Fausti V, Cozzani E, Cribier B, et al. Scleromyxedema: a multicenter study of characteristics, comorbidities, course, and therapy in 30 patients. J Am Acad Dermatol. 2013;69(1):66–72.
6. Santmyire-Rosenberger B, Dugan EM. Skin involvement in dermatomyositis. Curr Opin Rheumatol. 2003;15(6):714–22.

Chapter 10
A Middle-Aged Man Presenting with a New Asymmetrical Poikilodematous Erythema on the Lateral Neck

Paweł Pietkiewicz

Short Clinical Story of the Patient A 44y/o man visited the dermatology outpatients for a control visit. He had been treated for comedones on his back and retroauricular area 6 months ago, and he expressed his satisfaction with the treatment. He was advised to abstain from high glucose-index products, limit the carbohydrates and diary and was prescribed niacinamide (B3) 5 × 200 mg, riboflavin (B2) 3 × 6 mg for 2 months, yet he admitted to modify the dosage by himself to 2 × 200 mg and 2 × 3 mg, respectively. During the visit, an asymptomatic unilateral poikilodematous erythematous rash was noticed on his right neck, that he was not aware of (Fig. 10.1). The patient was Fitzpatrick III, had no history of concomitant diseases, was taking no other medications and reported no allergies. Medical investigation including his profession, hobbies, travels, history of sun-exposure, housing conditions, use of supplements, and perfumes, revealed no culprit factors. The medical examination was noncontributory and the patient did not report any other symptoms

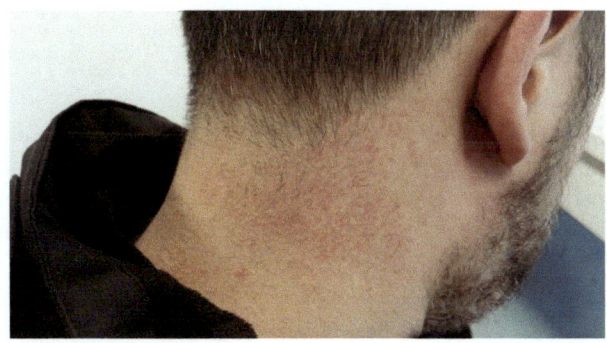

Fig. 10.1 Asymmetrical poikilodematous erythema on the lateral neck in a middle-aged man

P. Pietkiewicz (✉)
General and Oncological Surgery Clinic I, Greater Poland Cancer Center, Poznań, Poland

T. M. Lotti et al. (eds.), *Clinical Cases in Facial Erythema*, Clinical Cases in Dermatology, https://doi.org/10.1007/978-3-031-05996-4_10

Fig. 10.2 Dermatoscopy of the poikilodermatous erythema on the lateral neck in a middle-aged man (Dermlite DL4): Uniform reticular pattern formed by the linear vessels, pierced by the whitish hair follicle openings

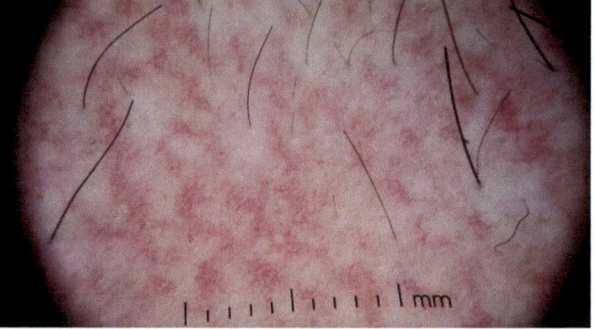

from any other systems. Dermatoscopy of the area affected showed the uniform pattern of reticular linear vessels pierced by the whitish hair follicle openings, which made the pattern polygonal. No evident white keratin plugs or pigmented structures were seen (Fig. 10.2).

Based on the Case Description and the Photographs, What Is Your Diagnosis?

- Erythemo-telangiectatic variant of poikiloderma of Civatte
- Poikilodermatous mycosis fungoides (PMF)
- Erythromelanosis follicularis faciei et colli (EFFC)
- Niacinamide-induced flushing

Diagnosis Niacinamide-induced flushing.

Discussion

Poikiloderma of Civatte is a relatively common idiopathic condition, usually developing in the fourth to seventh decade of life, mostly in post-menopausal woman and patients with fair skin types [1, 2]. The rash is symmetrical, and commonly both sides of the neck, lateral aspect of the cheeks, and anterior upper chest are affected, yet the skin under the chin remains spared as it is shaded from the sun, as the disease is sun-related [3]. The condition features skin atrophy, telangiectatic vessels and usually reddish-brownish hyperpigmentation [1]. The rash in abovementioned patient was unilateral, thus asymmetric. He had III skin type, and had no history of sun-exposure (as he was a remote worker at the time of COVID19 pandemic) or sun-damage. Dermatoscopy of poikiloderma of Civatte reveals mixed vascular pattern of dots, clods and linear serpentine vessels, spared perifollicular areas, and some follicular keratotic plugs [2].

PMF, formerly known as poikiloderma vasculare atrophicans or parapsoriasis variegate, is a rare, usually asymptomatic variant of cutaneous T-cell lymphoma [4]. Poikilodermatous hypo-hyperpigmented net-like atrophic and wrinkled erythematous patches or large plaques with telangiectatic vessels are commonly localized on the trunk and over the flexures. The presentation on a sun-unexposed area should be the clue to this entity [4]. However, the surface of the lesion in the described patient was smooth. Dermatoscopy of PMF usually feature grey-brown dots arranged in polygonal pattern, and dotted and looped vessels within this polygonal grid [5].

EFFC is a rare condition of unknown origin, manifesting as a bilateral, symmetrical brownish-reddish pigmentation, in some cases associated with keratosis pilaris [6, 7]. It commonly starts in childhood and adolescence. The classical rash is bilateral, yet there are single cases of unilateral distribution [8]. The disease was observed to present whitish scales, perifollicular blue-grey dots, and whitish follicular keratotic plugs over a reddish brown background in dermatoscopy [2].

Niacinamide-induced flushing is a common side effect in patients taking this drug, and the rash may be aggravated by alcohol [9]. It has a tendency toward self-limitation and can be controlled with anti-prostaglandin action of the nonsteroidal anti-inflammatory drugs (such as aspirin) [9]. In most cases, the tolerance to flushing develops over time [10], yet cessation of the drug is always enough to recover. The other symptoms, such as headache, lightheadedness, itching sensation, nausea and/or vomiting may be the heralds of vitamin B3 toxicity, yet the erythema itself is not associated with overdose [9]. The anti-comedogenic and anti-inflammatory properties of niacinamide led its' way to off-label use in acne, rosacea and seborrhea [11–13], yet the drug is a promising agent preventing cardiovascular events, premature aging, neurological disorders, and squamous cell carcinoma [14]. With its' wider use, physicians should consider it one of the possible triggers of head and neck erythema, that can be asymmetrical in distribution, and either asymptomatic or accompanied with burning or tingling sensation [9]. That is the first report of dermatoscopy of niacinamide-induced poikilodermatous erythema, with a vascular pattern distinct to the ones already known for clinically similar differential diagnoses. Further observations are needed in regard to specificity of that clue.

Key Points
- In patients with facial flushing/head-and-neck erythema, especially transient and asymmetrical, physicians should consider the role of niacinamide supplementation, as even non-toxic doses may evoke the symptoms.
- Dermatoscopy is a usable auxiliary diagnostic modality, that paired with taking the detailed history and clinical examination, may help to exclude some differentials and provide the dermatologist with the clues to the diagnosis.

References

1. Fernández-Nieto D, de Perosanz-Lobo D, Ortega-Quijano D, Jiménez-Cauhé J, Bea-Ardebol S. A typical red neck. Aust J Gen Pract. 2019 Aug;48(8):545–6.
2. Errichetti E, Stinco G. Dermoscopy in facilitating the recognition of Poikiloderma of Civatte. Dermatol Surg Off Publ Am Soc Dermatol Surg Al. 2018 Mar;44(3):446–7.
3. Katoulis AC, Stavrianeas NG, Georgala S, Bozi E, Kalogeromitros D, Koumantaki E, et al. Poikiloderma of Civatte: a clinical and epidemiological study. J Eur Acad Dermatol Venereol JEADV. 2005 Jul;19(4):444–8.
4. Pankratov O, Gradova S, Tarasevich S, Pankratov V. Poikilodermatous mycosis fungoides: clinical and histopathological analysis of a case and literature review. Acta Dermatovenerol Alp Pannonica Adriat. 2015;24(2):37–41.
5. Xu P, Tan C. Dermoscopy of poikilodermatous mycosis fungoides (MF). J Am Acad Dermatol. 2016 Mar 1;74(3):e45–7.
6. Maouni S, El Anzi O, Sqalli A, Znati K, Meziane M, Hassam B. Erythromelanosis follicularis faciei et colli: Dermoscopy and dermatopathology correlates. JAAD Case Rep. 2019 Jun 8;5(6):535–6.
7. Thielmann CM, Sondermann W. Erythromelanosis Follicularis Faciei et Colli: a case report in a Caucasian male and brief review of the literature. Case Rep Dermatol. 2020 Nov 16;12(3):231–5.
8. McGillis ST, Tuthill RJ, Ratz JL, Richards SW. Unilateral erythromelanosis follicularis faciei et colli in a young girl. J Am Acad Dermatol. 1991 Aug;25(2 Pt 2):430–2.
9. Habibe MN, Kellar JZ. Niacin Toxicity. In: StatPearls [Internet]. Treasure Island (FL): StatPearls Publishing; 2020 [cited 2021 Jan 29]. Available from: http://www.ncbi.nlm.nih.gov/books/NBK559137/
10. Kamanna VS, Ganji SH, Kashyap ML. The mechanism and mitigation of niacin-induced flushing. Int J Clin Pract. 2009 Sep;63(9):1369–77.
11. Gehring W. Nicotinic acid/niacinamide and the skin. J Cosmet Dermatol. 2004 Apr;3(2):88–93.
12. Walocko FM, Eber AE, Keri JE, Al-Harbi MA, Nouri K. The role of nicotinamide in acne treatment. Dermatol Ther. 2017 Sep;30(5)
13. Markovics A, Tóth KF, Sós KE, Magi J, Gyöngyösi A, Benyó Z, et al. Nicotinic acid suppresses sebaceous lipogenesis of human sebocytes via activating hydroxycarboxylic acid receptor 2 (HCA2). J Cell Mol Med. 2019 Sep;23(9):6203–14.
14. Djadjo S, Bajaj T. Niacin. In: StatPearls [Internet]. Treasure Island (FL): StatPearls Publishing; 2020 [cited 2021 Jan 29]. Available from: http://www.ncbi.nlm.nih.gov/books/NBK541036/

Chapter 11
A Middle-Aged Man with Erythema and Nodules on His Face

Runping Fang

A 48-year-old male farmer presented with erythema nodules on his face (Fig. 11.1a) and eyebrows falling off for half a year. A large number of nodules occurred in the face, limbs and trunk half a year ago. They were treated at the village health center and most of the nodules subsided. A large number of large red papular nodules appeared on both buttocks (Fig. 11.1b), limbs (Fig. 11.1c, d) and trunk due to unbroken diet half a month ago. Facial nodules and infiltration were obvious, and 1/3 of eyebrows fell off.

Based on the Case Description and the Photograph, What Is Your Diagnosis?

1. Neurofibromatosis
2. Nodular xanthomas
3. Leprosy
4. Seborrheic dermatitis

In the early stage of the patient, patchy lesions were found on the face, chest and back, with light red or light color and unclear boundary. Leprosy bacilli could be found in most tissues. The patients were treated with MDT-MB regimen and given 600 mg rifampicin in QD surveillance. Clofazimine 300 mg, QD surveillance and 50 mg QD self-administered; Dapsone 100 mg, self-administered Qd, for a course of 12 months.

R. Fang (✉)
Department of Dermatology, Shangyou County People's Hospital, Jiangxi Province, Ganzhou, China

© The Author(s), under exclusive license to Springer Nature
Switzerland AG 2022
T. M. Lotti et al. (eds.), *Clinical Cases in Facial Erythema*, Clinical Cases in
Dermatology, https://doi.org/10.1007/978-3-031-05996-4_11

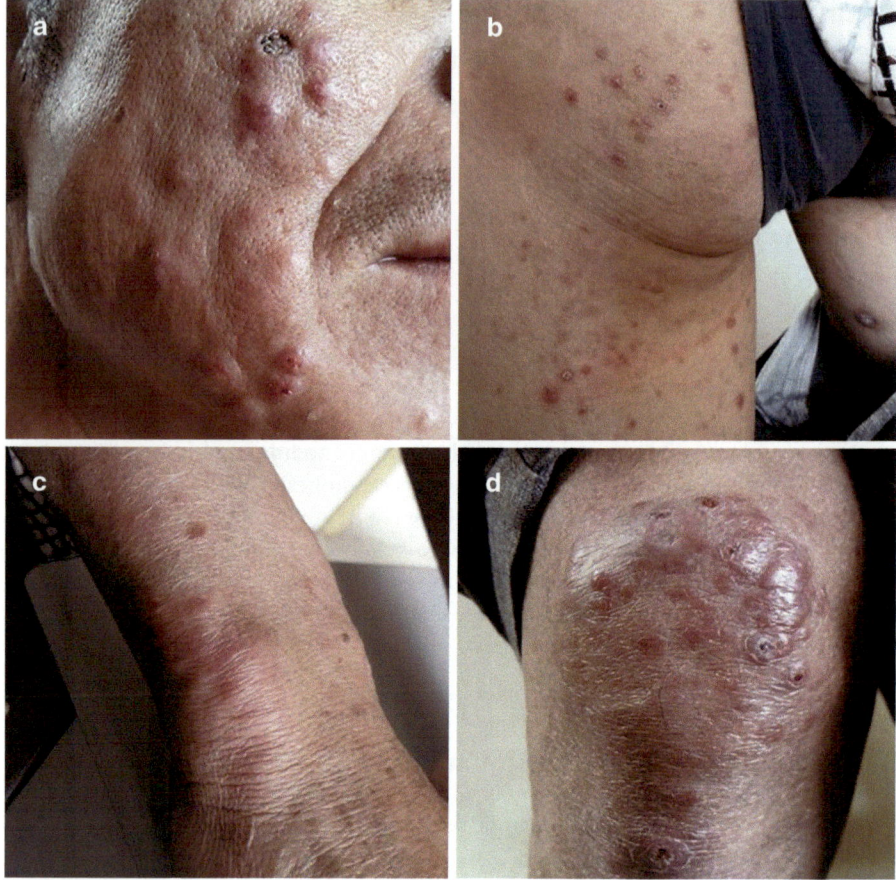

Fig. 11.1 Clinical manifestation of the patient. (**a**) erythematous nodule on his face; (**b**) A large number of erythematous papules can be seen on the buttocks, and some of them are necrotic in the center; (**c**) Red papule on forearm of hand; (**d**) Red macular papules on lower extremities

Histopathological examination showed that the tissue was covered with layered squamous epithelium, and there were a lot of histiocytes, foam cells, and lymphocytes in the subepithelium (Fig. 11.2).

Laboratory tests showed WBC 12.6×10^9/L, N 73%, ANA antibody spectrum was normal, TP and HIV were normal. Acid fast bacilli in skin tissue fluid smears showed: bacterial density index (BI) 3.0, left supraorbital 2+, right supraorbital 2+; left earlobe 3+, right earlobe 3+; mandibular 4+; right thigh lateral skin lesion 4+.

Diagnosis

Leprosy.

Fig. 11.2 There are macrophages and numerous foam cells in the dermis. (HE×20)

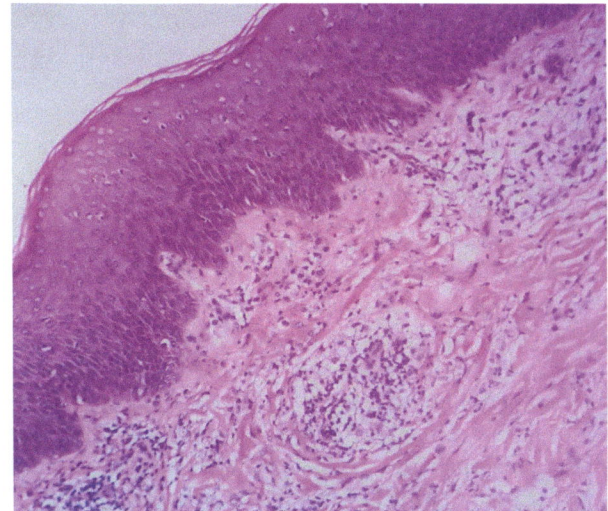

Discussion

Leprosy patients lack immunity to Mycobacterium leprae, and Mycobacterium leprae spreads all over the body through lymph and blood. Therefore, the range of invasion of tissues and organs is relatively wide. Skin lesion characteristics is large number, wide distribution and symmetry, blurred edges, tendency to fusion, and greasy and smooth surface. In addition to light spots, skin color mostly develops from red to reddish yellow and brownish yellow. The sensory disturbance is very light. In the early stage, the eyebrow and eyelashes began to fall from the outside of the eyebrow, and then the eyelashes also fell off, which is a clinical feature of leprosy. Leprosy bacilli test was strongly positive, skin lesions were macular, infiltration, nodules and diffuse damage. Early patchy lesions are distributed all over the body, especially on the face, chest and back. The color is light red or light, and the boundary is not clear. It should be carefully examined in good light before identification. After that, in addition to the increase of skin lesions, superficial and diffuse infiltrative nodules were formed. Because of infiltration and diffuse thickening of the face, the appearance of mild swelling, eyebrows and eyelashes often fall off. Later, the lesions fuse into large infiltrations, or nodules appear on the lesions and diffuse infiltrations. On the face, there are diffuse thickening, deepening dermatoglyphs, hypertrophy of nose and lip, enlargement of earlobe, loss of eyebrows and eyelashes, thinning or large shedding of hair, mixing of nodules and deep infiltration, congestion of conjunctiva, forming a "lion like" appearance. There are many nodules of different sizes in the extensor side of limbs, shoulder, back, buttock and scrotum. Later, due to diffuse damage, partial absorption, obvious sensory disturbance and sweating. In the lower leg, the skin is slightly hard, smooth and shiny, with fish-like or snake-like scale lesion, lasting for a long time. Some hair is almost naked, and residual hair is mostly distributed along the remaining blood vessels.

Although the neural stem was involved, the sensory disturbance was mild and the performance was late. The nerve trunk is slightly thick, symmetrical and soft, and muscular atrophy, deformity may occur in the late stage. The damage of nasal mucosa appeared earlier, hyperemia and swelling at first, then with the aggravation of the disease, nodules, infiltration and ulcer occurred. The lymph nodes were involved in the early stage, mild swelling, often not noticed by people. In the middle and late stage, the swelling was obvious, with tenderness. Testicular involvement, swelling at first, then atrophy, and tenderness, breast swelling and so on. Eye involvement can occur conjunctivitis, keratitis, iridocyclitis, etc. Internal organs are also involved, such as hepatosplenomegaly [1].

The clinical diagnosis of this disease is difficult, and the diagnosis mainly depends on histopathology. Microscopic examination revealed that the tissue was covered with multiple squamous epithelium, and numerous tissue cells, foam cells and lymphocyte aggregates were seen beneath the epithelium. The diagnosis can be made according to the typical clinical manifestations, histopathological and immunopathological features. But it should be differentiated from neurofibroma, nodular xanthomatosis, seborrheic dermatitis and other diseases.

Neurofibromatosis is an autosomal dominant disease in which a genetic defect causes the abnormal development of neural crest cells and leads to multi-system damage. According to the clinical manifestations and gene location can be divided into neurofibromatosis type I (NFI) and type II (NF II). The main features are cutaneous milk-coffee spots and peripheral nerve multiple neurofibromas [2].

Nodular xanthomas are flat yellow plaques or circular yellow papules, nodules or tumors. It is characterized by round, single or clustered yellow or orange nodules of different sizes, flat or high. It can occur in the joints of fingers and toes, armpit, groin, face, buttocks and mucous membrane. The early damage is bright yellow or red. Nodular xanthoma in the face should be differentiated from leprosy, and histopathology can be used for differentiation [3].

Seborrheic dermatitis is a kind of chronic inflammatory skin disease, which often occurs in areas with strong sebum secretion, such as head, face, chest, armpit, etc. The typical lesions are dark yellow red spots, patches or macular papules with clear edges, covered with greasy scales or crusts. Leprosy can be distinguished from acid-fast bacilli negative staining of the tissue fluid [4].

The detection of leprosy bacilli bacteria of Leprosy tumefaciens was strongly positive, 5–6+. Late reaction of leprosy test was negative. The cellular immune function test showed obvious defects. Early treatment can have a good prognosis, less deformity, late can cause disability. This type is relatively stable, only a few can be converted to BL under certain conditions.

Early, timely, sufficient, sufficient, regular treatment, can make the disease recovery faster, reduce deformity disability and recurrence. In order to reduce the occurrence of drug resistance, it is now advocated that several effective anti leprosy chemical drugs should be combined for treatment. Patients who have completed the combined chemotherapy should be monitored until the active symptoms completely disappear, and those who have positive skin smear should be checked once 3 months after the negative turn, If the skin smear is negative, it will be cured when the active symptoms disappear completely and the skin smear is still negative. The patient was followed up for 2 years without recurrence.

Key Points
- Leprosy is a disease with multiple morphological changes of skin lesions. The clinical manifestations of facial erythema, papules and nodules are easily confused with other diseases
- The key to the treatment of leprosy is early, timely, sufficient, full and standardized

References

1. Nascimento OJ. Leprosy neuropathy: clinical presentations. Arq Neuropsiquiatr. 2013;71(9B):661–6. https://doi.org/10.1590/0004-282X20130146.
2. Gerber PA, Antal AS, Neumann NJ, et al. Neurofibromatosis. Eur J Med Res. 2009;14(3):102–5. https://doi.org/10.1186/2047-783x-14-3-102.
3. Singh AP, Sikarwar S, Jatav OP, et al. Normolipemic tuberous xanthomas. Indian J Dermatol. 2009;54(2):176–9. https://doi.org/10.4103/0019-5154.53190.
4. Clark GW, Pope SM, Jaboori KA. Diagnosis and treatment of seborrheic dermatitis. Am Fam Physician. 2015;91(3):185–90.

Chapter 12
A Red Signal for Cancer

Ratnakar Shukla, Sharmila Patil, Aswathy Radhakrishan, and Anant Patil

Case Presentation

A 65 year old male married retired professional presented with history of swelling and redness of face since last 15 days. The swelling first appeared below left eye when the gradually spread to involve area around both eyes and rest of the face over next 2–3 days (Fig. 12.1).

Swelling over face was associated with itching. Swelling and redness of face appeared after application of hair dye. There was no history of raised lesions over body with recurrence. Swelling appeared over lips after few days of initial onset, but subsided on its own. There was no history of fever or difficulty in breathing or swallowing. Also, there was no history of hoarseness/change in voice. The patient gave history of increased swelling over face during daytime. There was no history of any drug intake, insect bite or topical application of medication. He had history of photosensitivity.

After 7–8 days of onset of swelling and redness of face, patient started developing painful lesions in the mouth with associated difficulty in eating solid food. He also started developing pain over fingers and difficulty in opening and closing movements (Fig. 12.2). There was no history of discoloration or intolerance to cold.

R. Shukla (✉)
Department of Dermatology, AIIMS-Gorakhpur, Gorakhpur, Uttar Pradesh, India

S. Patil
Department of Dermatology, AIIMS-Gorakhpur, Gorakhpur, Uttar Pradesh, India

Department of Dermatology, Dr. DY Patil School of Medicine, Nerul, Navi Mumbai, India

A. Radhakrishan
Department of Dermatology, Dr. DY Patil School of Medicine,
Nerul, Navi Mumbai, Maharashtra, India

A. Patil
Department of Pharmacology, Dr. DY Patil School of Medicine,
Nerul, Navi Mumbai, Maharashtra, India

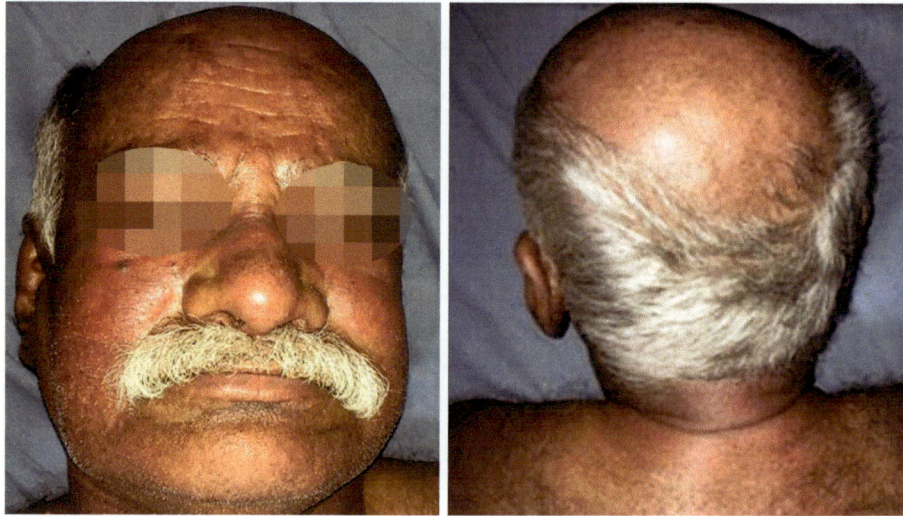

Fig. 12.1 Redness of face and back in the patient

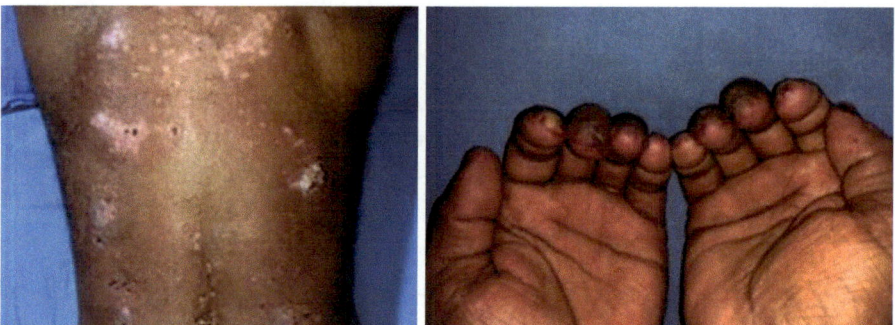

Fig. 12.2 Lesions on back and fingers

The patient had similar complaints 2 months back when he developed redness and swelling over face, neck, scalp, upper back (Fig. 12.2) and upper chest. He had history of joint pain (both elbows). There was no fever, proximal muscle weakness, breathlessness, cough, loss of appetite, fever, altered bowel habits, bleeding in stools or weight loss.

Cutaneous examination showed diffuse erythema on bilateral cheeks, periorbital area and scalp (Heliotrope rash), diffuse erythema over V-area of upper chest and neck (V-sign) and diffuse erythema on back of neck of upper back (Shawl sign). Mild scaling was present over face, neck and upper chest and back.

Oral cavity had 3, white color plaques on buccal mucosa. There were multiple crusted plaques and papules on bilateral elbow joints. Trunk examination showed multiple well defined erythematous papules over trunk. On back examination, multiple hypopigmented patches were seen (Fig. 12.2).

He had history of hypertension and type 2 diabetes mellitus for which he was taking treatment. Patient had history of smoking and drinking alcohol which he quitted about 15 years back.

No significant abnormality was observed on systemic examination. Based on the clinical examination, patient was provisionally diagnosed as allergic contact dermatitis secondary to hair dye application.

Based on the Case Description and the Photographs What Is Your Diagnosis?

- Dermatomyositis sine myositis
- Systemic Lupus Erythematosus
- Mixed connective tissue disorder

Laboratory investigations (Table 12.1) showed elevated levels of SGOT, LDH, C3, serum aldolase and CPK. Anti-Mi2, Anti-Ro, Anti-Jo1, Anti-DsDNA, Anti-Ku, Anti PM Scl, Anti Scl 70 and Anti U1RNP were negative. Chest X ray and abdominal ultrasound examination was normal.

Diagnosis: "Clinically Amyopathic Dermatomyositis"

He was treated with photoprotection and physical sunscreen. Pharmacological treatment included tablet prednisolone 40 mg once daily and tapered to 10 mg over 3 weeks. He was also treated with tablet hydroxychloroquine 200 mg twice daily, tablet azathioprine 50 mg once daily and tablet levocetirizine 5 mg once daily.

Table 12.1 Investigations

Laboratory parameter	Result
Haemoglobin (Hb)	13 mg/dL
SGOT	66 Units/L
Lactic acid dehydrogenase (LDH)	667.8 U/L
C3	236.5 mg/dL
C4	35.5 mg/dL
Erythrocyte sedimentation rate (ESR)	16 mm/h
C-reactive protein (CRP)	0.5 mg/dL
Serum aldolase	7.37 U/L
ANA	Weakly positive
Creatine phosphokinase (CPK)	214 mcg/L

Topical mometasone was advised for local application and tacrolimus gel for oral cavity was also given to this patient.

Treatment of hypertension (tablet amlodipine and ramipril) and diabetes (tablet metformin 500 mg once daily) was continued.

Follow Up

Four months after discharge, patient was contacted telephonically. He reported shortness of breath, weight-loss and cough. High-resolution computed tomography thorax showed centrally located masses extending into the lung parenchyma. Lung biopsy was suggestive of small cell lung carcinoma. He developed hepatomegaly. Liver biopsy showed metastatic poorly differentiated carcinoma. Immuno-histochemistry showed metastasis of small cell carcinoma of lung. The patient succumbed to lung carcinoma.

Discussion

Dermatomyositis is a chronic inflammatory disorder affecting skin and muscles. Patients often present with proximal muscle weakness and skin lesions. Muscle weakness is symmetrical [1]. Classic skin manifestations of DM include the helio-trope rash, Gottron's papules, Gottron's sign, the V-sign, and shawl sign [1].

We present a case of clinically amyopathic dermatomyositis, a type of dermato-myositis, with skin lesions suggestive of dermatomyositis with little or no evidence of myositis. Such cases constitute about 20% cases of dermatomyositis [2]. Diagnosis of amyopathic dermatomyositis may be challenging due to absence of classical muscle findings. Patients with clinically amyopathic dermatomyositis may have subclinical muscle disease [3]. Our patient did not have symmetrical muscle weakness. However other signs (heliotrope rash, V-sign, shawl sign) were classical presentation of dermatomyositis.

Usually, the condition is diagnosed based on the clinical examination and labora-tory investigations. Histopathology is useful for confirmation. However, in the pres-ence of only skin involvement in amyopathic dermatomyositis, histopathology is essential [4].

The treatment of dermatomyositis includes glucocorticoids and disease-modifying drugs [5]. Our patient was also treated with these drugs.

Dermatomyositis may be associated with different types of carcinomas. Dermatomyositis may be present before diagnosis of malignancy, both may present simultaneously or dermatomyositis may be observed after the diagnosis of malig-nancies. Association of breast, bladder and gastric carcinomas with dermatomyosi-tis has been reported in cases from India [6]. There is no significant difference in rates of carcinoma between clinically amyopathic dermatomyositis and classic dermatomyositis [2, 7]. Older age is associated significant risk of internal malignancy [7]. Severe skin disease, more severe muscular problems and dysphasia are other risk factors [1]. Our patient had presence of dysphasia and he succumbed to lung carcinoma. Considering common association, we feel, all patients with dermatomyositis should be evaluated for presence of malignancy. Moreover, clinicians should be familiar with clinically amyopathic dermatomyositis so that patients can be diagnosed early and accurately [3].

Key Points
- Clinically amyopathic dermatomyositis can be associated with carcinoma
- Elderly patients with dermatomyositis should be promptly and carefully evaluated.
- Evaluation methods include detail medical history, physical examination and relevant investigations
- Age appropriate screening for carcinoma should also be done in these patients

References

1. Marvi U, Chung L, Fiorentino DF. Clinical presentation and evaluation of dermatomyositis. Indian J Dermatol. 2012;57:375–81.
2. Sato S, Kuwana M. Clinically amyopathic dermatomyositis. Curr Opin Rheumatol. 2010;22:639–43.
3. Bailey EE, Fiorentino DF. Amyopathic dermatomyositis: definitions, diagnosis, and management. Curr Rheumatol Rep. 2014;16:465.
4. Sena P, Gianatti A, Gambini D. Dermatomyositis: clinicopathological correlations. G Ital Dermatol Venereol. 2018;153:256–64.
5. Jakubaszek M, Kwiatkowska B, Maślińska M. Polymyositis and dermatomyositis as a risk of developing cancer. Reumatologia. 2015;53:101–5.
6. Tambe SA, Jerajani HR. Dermatomyositis associated with malignancy: a report of 3 cases. Indian Dermatol Online J. 2013;4:326–32.
7. Leatham H, Schadt C, Chisolm S, Fretwell D, Chung L, Callen JP, Fiorentino D. Evidence supports blind screening for internal malignancy in dermatomyositis: data from 2 large US dermatology cohorts. Medicine (Baltimore). 2018;97(2):e9639.

Chapter 13
A Woman with Facial Butterfly Erythema

Wen-Jia Yang, Hao Guo, Tian-Hua Xu, Xing-Hua Gao, and Jiu-Hong Li

A 57-year-old woman presented to the department with her complaining of the butterfly erythema on bilateral cheeks (Fig. 13.1a, b) after picking her nose for 4 days. She also had pain in the skin lesions. She was also accompanied by fever and the highest body temperature was 38.9 °C. She was administered by azithromycin tablets, but with no obvious improvement.

Based on the Case Description and the Photograph, What Is Your Diagnosis?

1. Skin infections (erysipelas or cellulitis)
2. Autoimmune diseases (Systemic lupus erythematosus)
3. Contact dermatitis
4. Angioedema

She was hospitalized for further examination and treatment. The skin could be palpated with tenderness, tense and increased local skin temperature. A complete blood count showed a white blood cell (WBC) count of 2.47×10^9/L (3.5–9.5×10^9/L), granulocyte count of 1.15×10^9/L (1.8–6.3×10^9/L). laboratory tests showed elevated serum C-reactive protein (CRP) 9.3 mg/L (0–5 mg/L)

W.-J. Yang · H. Guo (✉) · X.-H. Gao · J.-H. Li
Department of Dermatology, The First Hospital of China Medical University, Shenyang, China

T.-H. Xu
Department of Dermatology, Shenzhen Nanshan Hospital, Shenzhen, China

T. M. Lotti et al. (eds.), *Clinical Cases in Facial Erythema*, Clinical Cases in Dermatology, https://doi.org/10.1007/978-3-031-05996-4_13

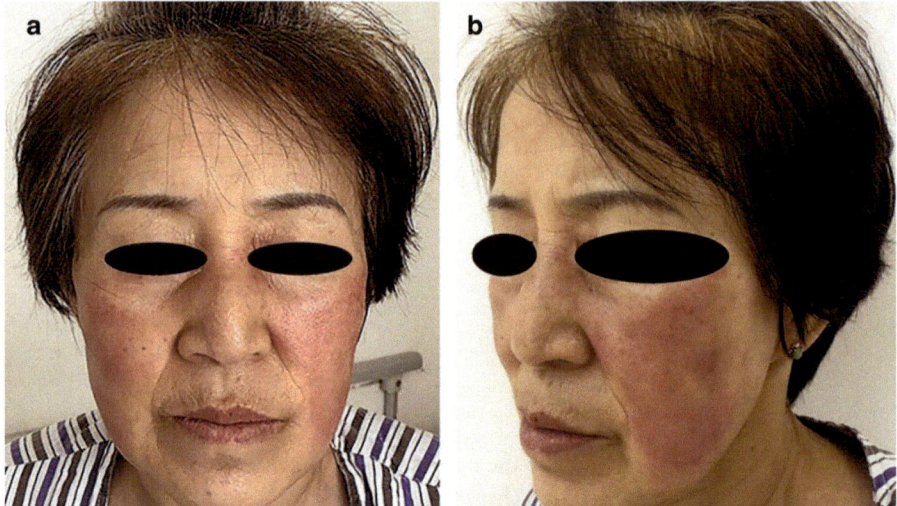

Fig. 13.1 (**a, b**) Clinical manifestation of the patient: well circumscribed and swollen erythema was noted on facial anteroposterior (**a**) and lateral (**b**) views

and erythrocyte sedimentation rate (ESR) 32 mm/h (15–20 mm/h). T-cell subgroup analysis showed that CD3, CD4 and CD8 cells values were lower than normal [CD3: 522/UL, (690–2540/UL), CD8: 154/UL (190–1140/UL), CD4: 351/UL (410–1590/UL)], but the proportion of the three was normal. The old lady had been with sero-positive (rheumatoid factor 62.9 IU/mL) rheumatoid arthritis (RA) for 20 years and was treated with leflunomide (20 mg once daily) for 2 months. Test for the possibility of systemic autoimmune diseases showed: complement levels, immunoglobulins, anticardiolipin antibodies, antinuclear antibodies (ANA), anti-double-stranded-DNA antibodies (dsDNA) and antineutrophil cytoplasmic antibodies (ANCA) were all normal. Test for syphilis and HIV were normal. Ultrasonic Doppler indicates thickening of dermis and subcutaneous tissue with echo enhancement.

The patient was given cefamandole in a dose of two gram by intravenous drip infusion two times a day. The facial erythema and swelling significantly relieved in 5 days.

Diagnosis

Erysipelas.

Discussion

Erysipelas is a skin infection of the superficial cutaneous lymphatics and upper dermis layer, which mainly caused by β-haemolytic streptococcal (BHS) [1]. BHS invades through the rupture of the skin or mucous membrane, and the infection is manifested as a well-defined erythema, and accompanied by local symptoms such as burning sensation, tenderness and itching. Tinea pedis and rhinitis are important risk factors for erysipelas in lower legs and face. People with diabetes, obesity and immunosuppression are susceptible to infection [2]. Erysipelas usually occurs unilaterally. However bilateral facial erysipelas is also common due to the loose subcutaneous tissue.

Erysipelas progresses rapidly after the onset of illness, often with prodromal symptoms such as fever, headache, nausea and vomiting, accompanied by typical skin lesions. Skin infections can manifest as systemic inflammatory response syndrome (SIRS), which two or more of the following criteria can be defined: (1) white blood cells $>12 \times 10^9$/L or $<4 \times 10^9$/L, (2) temperature >38 °C or <36 °C, (3) tachypnea >20 breaths/min, (4) heart rate >90 beats/min [3]. Improper treatment may cause serious local complications, such as local suppuration, necrosis or hemorrhagic purpura.

Antibiotics should be selected according to the results of bacterial culture of serum or local secretions, as well as the result of drug sensitivity test. Beta—lactam antibiotics are the first choice for treatment [4]. Generally, the body temperature can return to normal after 2–3 days of general medication, but the medication still needs to be continued for about 2 weeks. Severe patients may need longer treatment period. Some studies have shown that inappropriate use of antibiotics [2] and higher ESR are independent risk factors for developing local complications and higher chance of recurrent erysipelas.

After adequate course of appropriate antibiotic therapy, slight pigmentation and scales may be left on the surface of the skin lesions.

If the treatment is improper, the infection may further spread to the deep dermis and subcutaneous tissues and cause cellulitis. If it continues to progress, it will lead to complications such as fasciitis, subcutaneous abscess, cavernous sinus phlebitis, meningitis and death in severe cases.

The difference between erysipelas and cellulitis is that the latter is the infection of deeper subcutaneous tissue. The skin lesions of cellulitis are unclear, and there is a tendency for purulent inflammation. Erysipelas and cellulitis sometimes cannot make a clear diagnosis. Some scholars believe that they are the same disease [5].

Autoimmune connective tissue disease may present with facial erythema wich characterized by photosensitivity. Systemic lupus erythematosus may manifest with a butterfly erythema. Serum biochemical test show that ANA and ds DNA are positive. The skin manifestations of dermatomyositis (DM) are appeared with red and swollen erythema on cheeks and eyelids. The diagnosis of DM also based on elevation serum muscle enzymes and evidence of muscle damage [6].

Contact dermatitis has a history of exposure to external irritants. The skin lesions are mostly limited to the parts of direct contact. The systemic symptoms are small and the lesions can subside after stopping contact.

Angioedema is a transient and spontaneous edema of the subcutaneous and submucosal tissues. Swelling of the face, eyelids and lips often occurs, usually asymmetrically distributed. Acquired angioedema occurs in individuals with allergies. Hereditary angioedema leads to abnormal activation of C1 and decomposition from C2 to bradykinin due to the lack or inactivity of C1 esterase inhibitor (C1INH) [6]. Bradykinin is a substance that increases vascular permeability and causes tissue edema.

After 14 days of treatment, the lesions subsided, leaving post-inflammatory hyperpigmentation. Review the blood routine test and biochemical tests showed normal white blood cell count and CRP levels. The patient was followed up for 5 months without recurrence.

Key Points
- Erysipelas and cellulitis are a group of acute bacterial infectious skin diseases involving the deep layers of the cutaneous and subcutaneous tissues.
- Adequate and effective antibiotic treatment can relieve systemic symptoms, control the spread of inflammation and prevent recurrence.

References

1. Rath E, Skrede S, Mylvaganam H, Bruun T. Aetiology and clinical features of facial cellulitis: a prospective study. Infect Dis (Lond). 2018;50(1):27–34.
2. Dalal A, Eskin-Schwartz M, Mimouni D, et al. Interventions for the prevention of recurrent erysipelas and cellulitis. Cochrane Database Syst Rev. 2017;6:CD009758.
3. Corey GR, Wilcox MH, Gonzalez J, et al. Ceftaroline fosamil therapy in patients with acute bacterial skin and skin-structure infections with systemic inflammatory signs: a retrospective dose comparison across three pivotal trials. Int J Antimicrob Agents. 2019;53(6):830–7.
4. Russo A, Concia E, Cristini F, et al. Current and future trends in antibiotic therapy of acute bacterial skin and skin-structure infections. Clin Microbiol Infect. 2016;22:S27–36.
5. Stevens DL, Bisno AL, Chambers HF, et al. Practice guidelines for the diagnosis and management of skin and soft tissue infections: 2014 update by the infectious diseases society of America. Clin Infect Dis. 2014;59(2):147–59.
6. Batista M, Goncalo M. The rash that presents as a red swollen face. Clin Dermatol. 2020;38(1):63–78.

Chapter 14
An Elderly Female with Lacy, Reticulated and White Streaks

Bing-Yan Yang, Nan Yu, and Yong-Long Gao

An 51-year-old female presented to the outpatient with her daughter and complaining of Slacy, reticulated and white streaks on her Lips for the past 1 years (Fig. 14.1).

Based on the Case Description and the Photograph, What Is Your Diagnosis?

1. Lichen planus
2. Leukoplakia
3. Candidiasis
4. Pemphigus

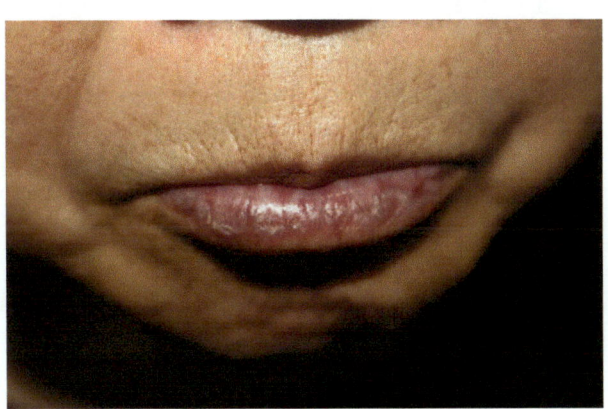

Fig. 14.1 An 51-year-old female presented complaining of Slacy, reticulated and white streaks on her Lips for the past 1 years

B.-Y. Yang · N. Yu (✉) · Y.-L. Gao
Department of Dermatology, General Hospital of Ningxia Medical University, Yinchuan, Ningxia, China

© The Author(s), under exclusive license to Springer Nature Switzerland AG 2022
T. M. Lotti et al. (eds.), *Clinical Cases in Facial Erythema*, Clinical Cases in Dermatology, https://doi.org/10.1007/978-3-031-05996-4_14

Diagnosis

Lichen planus.

Discussion

Lichen planus is a papulosquamous disorder of debatable etiology, characterized by the formation of flat topped, polygonal greyish white, purple/lilac eruptions. Middle age people of both the sexes are its victims.

Its precise etiology is unknown. However, it may either be bacterial or viral in origin. Immunologic factors are also incriminated. It may also follow bone marrow transplantation or graft versus host reaction. Furthermore, certain individuals are genetically predisposed to it. Also several drugs such as chloroquine, quinacrine, streptomycin, paraaminio salicylic acid (PAS), methyldopa, quinidine, phenothiazine, chlorpropamide, gold, bismuth, levamisole, and penicillamine are incriminated. Exposure to paraphenylenediamine salts encountered in color photographic developermay also produce these lesions.

Mucosal surfaces are involved in nearly half the patients. The buccal mucosa and the tongue are most frequently affected. The mucosal lesions consist of lacy, reticulated, white streaks, papules, plaques, and erosions. Chronic erosive oral lichen planus may predispose to squamous cell carcinoma. Nearly 25% of the male patients have involvement of genitalia.

The diagnosis of lichen planus is clinical; however, it may be supplemented by histopathology. Hematoxylin-eosin stained section reveals the presence of: (1) Hyperkeratosis, (2) Focal hypergranulosis, (3) irregular acanthosis resulting in saw tooth appearance of rete ridges, (4) Liquefaction degeneration of basal cell layer, (5) A band like upper dermal lymphocytic infiltrate, (6) Incontinence of the melanin, (7) Colloid bodies may be present in the deep dermis, (8) Small separation between dermis and epidermis may be present (Max Joseph spaces) [1].

Currently there is no effective treatment method, more comprehensive treatment is used.

Key Points
- Lichen planus is a papulosquamous disorder of debatable etiology.
- An Elderly Female with lacy, reticulated and white streaks
- The diagnosis of lichen planus is clinical; however, it may be supplemented by histopathology.

Reference

1. Sehgal VN. Dermatovenereology. Beijing: Qinghua University Public; 2015. p. 96–100.

Chapter 15
An Intriguing Case of Red Face

Elena Mirceska Arsovska and Katerina Damevska

A 42-year-old female patient, presented to the clinic with facial skin lesions that are persisting for a couple of years. The patient has a history of psoriasis vulgaris that has been treated with topical, class 3 corticosteroids. She reports that 3–4 years ago, she started to apply the same corticosteroids preparations on her face, trying to treat her facial erythema.

Dermatological examination showed plaque psoriasis on the predilection sites of the body, with a BSA less than 5%. In addition, marked facial erythema and telangiectasia especially over the cheeks and nose, papules and few pustules, hirsutism and atrophy with hypopigmentation just above the right lower vermilion (Figs. 15.1 and 15.2). The diagnosis of topical steroid damaged skin was established.

What Is the Best Treatment for the Patient?

1. Discontinuation of topical steroids
2. Treatment with low potent steroids
3. Treatment with calcineurin inhibitors
4. Systemic corticosteroids
5. Personalized treatment plan

E. Mirceska Arsovska · K. Damevska (✉)
Faculty of Medicine, University Clinic for Dermatology, Ss Cyril and Methodius University, Skopje, Macedonia

© The Author(s), under exclusive license to Springer Nature Switzerland AG 2022
T. M. Lotti et al. (eds.), *Clinical Cases in Facial Erythema*, Clinical Cases in Dermatology, https://doi.org/10.1007/978-3-031-05996-4_15

Fig. 15.1 Facial erythema, telangiectasias (red arrow), hypopigmentation and skin atrophy (blue arrow) in patient with topical steroid damaged skin

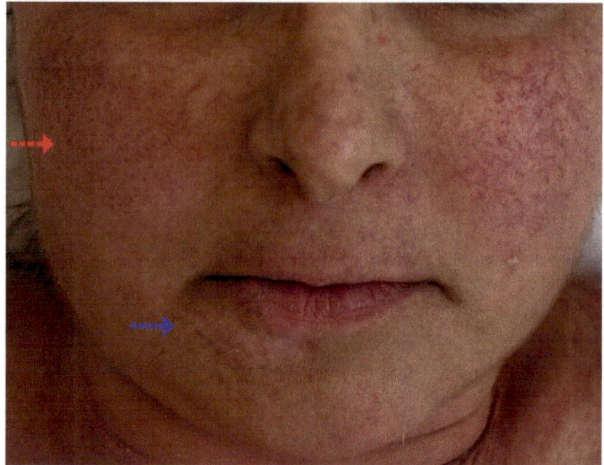

Fig. 15.2 Facial erythema, pustule (yellow arrow), hypopigmentation and skin atrophy (blue arrow) and hirsutism (black arrow) in patient with topical steroid damaged skin

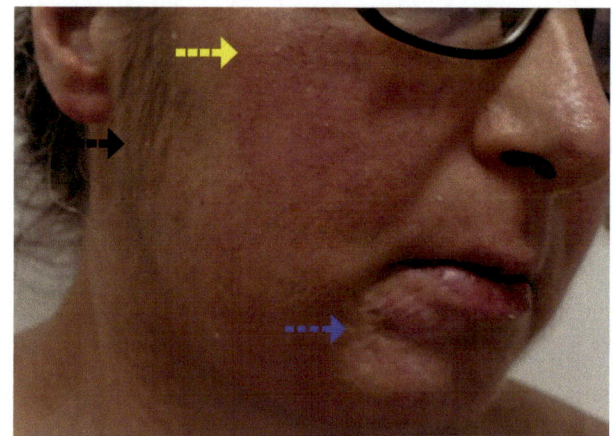

Answer

Personalized treatment plan.

Discussion

Topical corticosteroids (TC) first introduced in 1952, by Sulzberger and Witten [1], with wide range of potency from low to extremely high, are one of the most useful drugs for the treatment of dermatological disorders if used for the proper indication and duration. Anti-inflammatory, immunosuppressive, anti-proliferative and vaso-constrictive mechanisms responsible for their wanted are also responsible for their side effects if they are use in an improper way [2, 3].

Misapplication of TC, especially over the face, is prevalent worldwide. The face is the most commonly and severely affected site of such misuse because of increased penetrability due to the thinness of the skin of the face. Hence, for proper indication, only TCs of the least potency should be applied on the skin of the face. The duration should not go beyond 2 weeks, with once-daily application along with proper amount based on fingertip unit [4].

In addition to the common TCs adverse effects, their misuse on the face is manifested with new facial dermatoses: steroid rosacea, acneiform eruption, hypertrichosis and demodicidosis. The most severe adverse effect being "topical steroid damaged/dependent face" (TSDF) also named as "steroid addiction", "dermatitis rosaceaformis steroidica" or "red face syndrome" by different authors. TSDF is defined as semi-permanent or permanent damage to the skin of the face precipitated by the irrational, arbitrary, unsubstantiated, or prolonged use of TCs resulting in a plethora of cutaneous signs and symptoms and psychological dependence to the drug [5].

Clinical features of TSDF are erythema, papules, pustules, acneiform eruptions, hirsutism, telangiectasia, tinea incognito, hypo- and hyper-pigmentation, perioral dermatitis, rosacea-like features, allergic contact dermatitis, photosensitivity, atrophy, and striae. Attempts to withdraw the drug result in a flare of symptoms causing significant distress to the patient prompting resumption of TC's usage and refusal of any further trials to withdraw the drug. The withdrawal of the TCs has a cyclic flare pattern (rebound phenomenon), that initially results in mild erythema at the site of the original lesion (red face) within a week of discontinuation, lasting for about 2 weeks, ending with desquamation. This rebound phenomenon may sometimes occur in an area larger than the original site of TC misapplication or even at distant sites. If the patient does not use the TC again, the flare resolves but reappears within 2 weeks. This pattern of flare and resolution repeats itself with shorter duration of flares and prolonged periods of resolution until the patient is completely cured. The duration of the withdrawal phase is correlated to length of TCs treatment [6].

Functional and anatomic cutaneous changes are underlying the pathogenesis of the clinical signs and symptoms of TSDF. Topical steroids may inhibit collagen synthesis, leading to dermal atrophy. Telangiectasises and background erythema result from the passive dilation of blood vessels and easier visualization of dermal capillaries because of the reduction in supporting connective tissue. Localized hypopigmentation may occur from inhibition of the function of melanocytes. The mechanism of how steroids promote vellus hair growth resulting in localized hypertrichosis is still unknown. The immunosuppressive effects of topical steroids may facilitate the overgrowth of various bacteria, yeast, demodex mites, or other microorganisms in pilosebaceous glands, resulting in inflammatory reactions that produce papules and pustules. These microorganisms may subsequently act as superantigens, causing an immunologic response with an accompanying proinflammatory cytokine release. Steroids also inhibit the release of endothelium-derived relaxing factor, a natural vasodilator. Vasoconstriction leads to a buildup of multiple metabolites, such as nitric oxide (a potent vasodilator) that leads to vasodilatation after discontinuation of steroids. As a result, the diameter of blood vessels enlarges beyond their original presteroid diameter, which potentiates the erythema, burning sensations, and pruritus seen in TSDF [7].

The treatment of TSDF requires long-term therapeutic management of both the rebound phenomenon and reversal of damage caused by the TC. The first and most essential step in the treatment is discontinuation of all topical steroids. However, whether this should be tapered or abrupt has not been determined. Japanese reports suggest minimal difference in the outcome and recommend immediate cessation [8, 9]. Patients must be counseled on the signs and symptoms of rebound phenomenon and informed on the slow disease regression, even after the exogenous factors have been removed and the appropriate treatments implemented. Without any treatment, the severity of the initial rebound tends to subside after 10–14 days. However, to avoid the rebound phenomenon of TC discontinuation, and/or to decrease its severity, patients can gradually taper the frequency of topical steroid applications, or switch to intermittent use of topical hydrocortisone 1% before discontinuation of all topical steroids. Goldman, [10], has found that varying doses (20–60 mg) of prednisone, tapered over 1–2 weeks at most, can be helpful in treating the initial flare-ups of TSDF. Replacement therapy with calcineurin inhibitors has been advocated by some workers. Topical calcineurin antagonists may offer quicker initial improvement and more rapid eventual resolution. Oral antihistamines and/or topical antipruritic agents, also can be prescribed for symptomatic relief of pruritus associated with the rebound phenomenon. In cases of intense burning sensation repeated ice compresses can be used. Bland emollients for the dryness and Burrow's solution for weepy lesions can also be used. Some investigators encourage patients to wash their face with water only and to abandon the use of all cosmetics, soaps, moisturizers, lotions, astringents, and day and night creams. The use of sunscreen is recommended in cases of photosensitivity. The rebound phenomenon and flares may have strong psychological impact on patients and difficulty dealing with discontinuation of topical steroid that requires emotional support from the dermatologists. Oral tetracyclines and low-dose isotretinoin can be used to treat steroid rosacea and perioral/periorificial dermatitis. Prevention or treatment of secondary infection may also require oral antibiotics. It is unknown if their antibacterial or anti- inflammatory effects are primarily responsible for the clinical benefit. The preferred oral antibiotics are lipophilic tetracyclines, such as doxycycline and minocycline, in dosages of 100–200 mg daily for 3–4 months. Longer duration of treatment is rarely needed. Oral metronidazole also has been used in patients who are unable to tolerate tetracyclines. If there is no improvement with a full dose of tetracycline, treatment with low-dose isotretinoin is an alternative. An average dose of 2–5 mg daily (often given as a 10-mg dose 2 or 3 times weekly) for 3 months has been found to be effective. In addition to oral antibiotics, topical clindamycin, erythromycin, metronidazole, sodium sulfacetamide 10% and sulfur 5% lotion can be used as part of the treatment regimen. Oral antifungals have also been used to control the resulting demodex/pityrosporum folliculitis in most of the cases [11].

Telangiectasia and hypertrichosis can be treated with laser. Stretch marks can also be treated with laser, platelet reach plasma (prp), skin needing or dermabrasion, but few have been proven to be effective.

The duration of acute topical corticosteroid withdrawal is variable from days to months, before eventually the skin becomes 'normal'. It can take weeks to years to return to its original condition. Given the above-mentioned consequences of undue TC use on the face and the long and lengthy process of their discontinuation, prevention is the best option, rising awareness for the patients and doctors of the risks and avoiding prolonged and unnesesery use of topical steroids.

Key Points
- TC is one of the most useful drugs in dermatology if they are used for proper indication and duration.
- Inappropriate use of TC can lead to many side effects and severe physiological addiction—topical steroid damaged/dependent face.
- Treatment of side effects and addiction in patients who misused TC is a complex and long-lasting process.

References

1. Sulzberger MB, Witten VH. The effect of topically applied compound F in selected dermatoses. J Invest Dermatol. 1952;19(2):101–2. https://doi.org/10.1038/jid.1952.72.
2. Hengge UR, Ruzicka T, Schwartz RA, Cork MJ. Adverse effects of topical glucocorticosteroids. J Am Acad Dermatol. 2006;54(1):1–18. https://doi.org/10.1016/j.jaad.2005.01.010.
3. Fisher DA. Adverse effects of topical corticosteroid use [published correction appears in West J Med 1995 May;162(5):476]. West J Med. 1995;162(2):123–6.
4. Saraswat A. Ethical use of topical corticosteroids. Indian J Dermatol. 2014;59(5):469–72. https://doi.org/10.4103/0019-5154.139877.
5. Lahiri K, Coondoo A. Topical steroid damaged/dependent face (TSDF): an entity of cutaneous pharmacodependence. Indian J Dermatol. 2016;61(3):265–72. https://doi.org/10.4103/0019-5154.182417.
6. Rapaport MJ, Lebwohl M. Corticosteroid addiction and withdrawal in the atopic: the red burning skin syndrome. Clin Dermatol. 2003;21(3):201–14. https://doi.org/10.1016/s0738-081x(02)00365-6.
7. Coondoo A, Phiske M, Verma S, Lahiri K. Side-effects of topical steroids: a long overdue revisit. Indian Dermatol Online J. 2014;5(4):416–25. https://doi.org/10.4103/2229-5178.142483.
8. Fukaya M, Sato K, Sato M, et al. Topical steroid addiction in atopic dermatitis. Drug Healthc Patient Saf. 2014;6:131–8. https://doi.org/10.2147/dhps.s6920.
9. Katoh N, Ohya Y, Ikeda M, et al. Japanese guidelines for atopic dermatitis 2020. Allergol Int. 2020;69(3):356–69. https://doi.org/10.1016/j.alit.2020.02.006.
10. Goldman D. Tacrolimus ointment for the treatment of steroid-induced rosacea: a preliminary report. J Am Acad Dermatol. 2001;44(6):995–8. https://doi.org/10.1067/mjd.2001.114739.
11. Chen AY, Zirwas MJ. Steroid-induced rosacealike dermatitis: case report and review of the literature. Cutis. 2009;83(4):198–204.

Chapter 16
An Old Women with Erythema, Pimples and Pain over Neck, Waist and Abdomen

Xiao-Dong Li, Juan Chen, Hao Guo, and Xing-Hua Gao

A 75-year-old women presented with multiple erythema, grouped pimples on right waist and abdomen (T9, L2) and on left side of armpit (T2, 3) for last 10 days. Previously, the patient had prodromal pain in the areas of skin involvement. His sleep was disturbed due to pain in the lesions. The patient was acutely ill-looking in appearance. She had previous gallbladder stones and fatty liver. On cutaneous examination, with erythema and grouped pimples were seen on the right of waist and abdomen (Fig. 16.1a, b showing in the T9, L2 nerve dermatome on the right side of waist and abdomen) and the left side of armpit (Fig. 16.1c showing in T2, 3 dermatome on the left side of the armpit).

Based on the Case Description and the Photograph, What Is Your Diagnosis?

1. Herpes hoster
2. Acute abdomen
3. Myocardial infarction

X.-D. Li (✉) · J. Chen
Department of Dermatology, Central Hospital Affiliated to Shenyang Medical College, Shenyang, China

H. Guo · X.-H. Gao
Department of Dermatology, The First Hospital of China Medical University, Shenyang, China

© The Author(s), under exclusive license to Springer Nature Switzerland AG 2022
T. M. Lotti et al. (eds.), *Clinical Cases in Facial Erythema*, Clinical Cases in Dermatology, https://doi.org/10.1007/978-3-031-05996-4_16

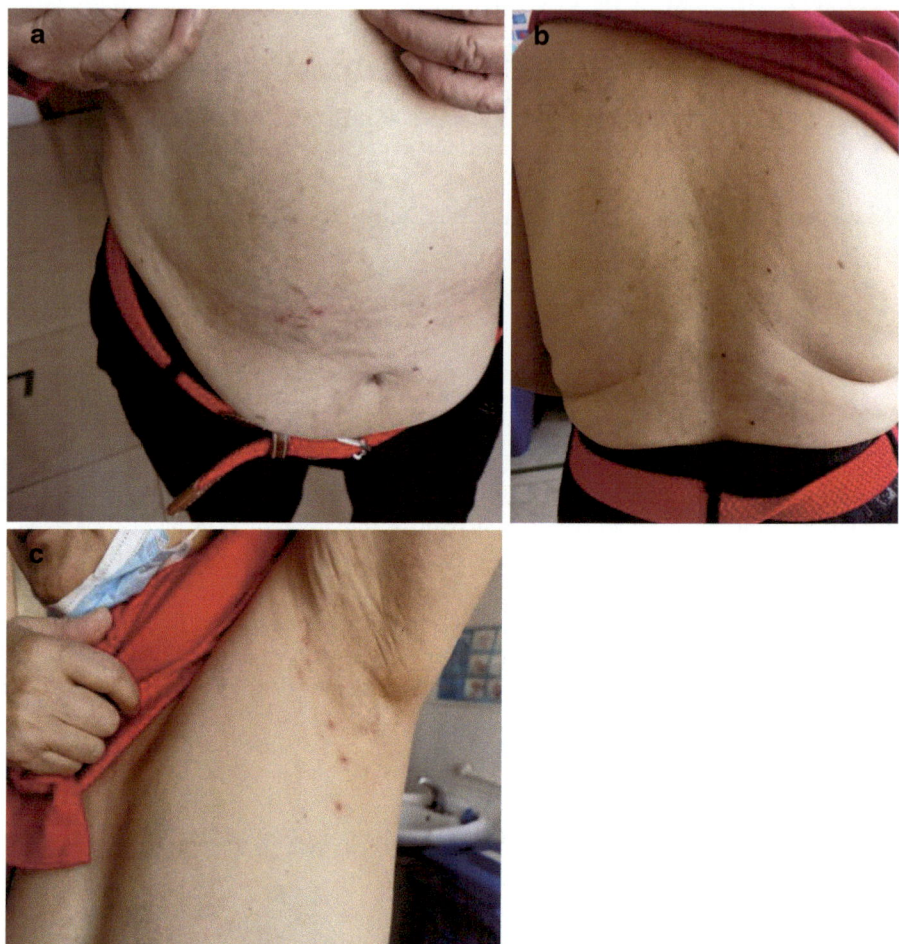

Fig. 16.1 (**a, b**) Showing in the T9, L2 nerve dermatome on the right side of waist and abdomen. (**c**) Showing in T2, 3 dermatome on the left side of the armpit

Because the patient has obvious symptoms of neuralgia,we treat it as herpes zoster based on our experience. He was treated with injection I/V Foscarnet sodium 2.0 g/day and with injection I/V Vitamin B to repair nerves. Pain was treated by pregabalin every 12 h, 2 times daily and tramadol 325 mg/day. Because of the severe pain, we used glucocorticoids to control the condition. The eruptions remained confined to the involved dermatome without any systemic involvement or spread. Cutaneous lesions healed gradually over a period of 10 days.

Abdominal ultrasound showed Fatty liver, liver cysts, gallbladder stones. The serum muscle enzyme tests, Blood routine, ECG, Chest radiograph were normal or negative. The erythrocyte sedimentation rate (ESR) was 10 mm/h (normal range 0–20 mm/h).

Diagnosis

Herpes Zoster Duplex Bilateralis.

Discussion

Herpes zoster duplex, simultaneous reactivation of VZV involving two different dermatomes, of which Herpes Zoster Duplex Unilateralis (HZDU), occurs unilaterally in two non-contiguous dermatomes while in Herpes Zoster Duplex Bilateralis (HZDB) it may occur in same (symmetric) or different dermatomes (asymmetric) bilaterally [1, 2]. We found all over the world reported dozens of cases of Herpes Zoster Duplex Bilateralis. Herpes zoster duplex bilateralis is an atypical presentation of herpes zoster that is usually found in patients with compromised immunity or in patients with advancing age. But Herpes Zoster Duplex Bilateralis is also reported in immuno-competent patients [3].The following are documents that had published previously (Table 16.1).The pathogenesis of herpes zoster duplex bilateralis needs further study.

Key Points
- Herpes Zoster Duplex Bilateralis, it is almost restricted to the immunocompromised patient. Occasionally affect healthy people.
- All over the world has reported dozens of cases of Herpes Zoster Duplex Bilateralis. It needs further study.

Table 16.1 Clinico-epidemiological overview of reported cases of herpes zoster duplex bilateralis

S. no	Country	Age/ sex	Dermatomes	Underlying disease	Year
1	China	52/F	L:T8 R:T2–3	Systemic lupus erythematosus	1971
2	/	67/M	L:V1–2 R:V3	None	1986
3	UK	76/F	L:V3 R:V1	None	1986
4	Japan	77/M	L:S3–4 R:T6–8	Stomach cancer	1989
5	USA	37/F	L:T11 R:T3	Asthma	1990
6	South Korea	5/F	L:T2 R:T5	None	1994
7	South Korea	10/M	L:L2–4 R:C4–6	HIV	1995
8	India	73/F	L:T9–10 R:L2–3,S3	Hemophilia	2001
9	Hungary	4/F	L:T5 R:T7–8	None	2001
10	Germany	16/F	L:T4–7 R:V2	None	2001
11	India	24/F	L:Eyes R: thighs	None	2002
12	South Korea	47/F	L:L3–4 R:T7	None	2004
13	Japan	72/F	L:Face R:calf	Diabetes	2007
14	Arab	64/F	L:T8 R:L4	Diabetes; polymyositis	2007
15	South Korea	67/F	L:T7–8 R:L4–5	Hypertension, osteoporosis	2009
16	France	64/F	L:C4 R:Eyes	Rheumatoid arthritis	2011
17	India	45/M	L:T9 R:Trigeminal nerve	None	2012
18	Belgium	70/M	L:L1–2 R:C4,T2	Leukemia	2012
19	Japan	61/M	L:C5,T1 R:T2–3	None	2013
20	India	26/M	L:T9 R:T8	None	2015
21	India	28/M	L:T12,L1–2 R:T8–9	None	2015
22	Japan	68/F	L:T4 R:T7–8	Multiple myeloma	2016
23	USA	3/F	L:T2–3 R:T2–3	Leukemia	1985
24	/	70/M	L:L1–2 R:C4,T2	Leukemia	2009
25	/	36/F	R:V1 L:Iliopinginal	/	/
26	/	55/M	L:L1,2 & S3,4 R:L1,2,3&S3	/	/
27	/	60/M	V1-R/L	None	1996
28	/	39/F	T8-R/L	Pancreatitis, diabetes, laparoscopic surgery	2006
29	/	75/M	V1-R/L	Prostate cancer	2002
30	/	30/M	T-10-R/L	HIV	2008
31	China	60/F	L:T3–4 R:T3–4	Tuberculosis	2016
32	China	64/F	L:C2 R:L1	Hypertension, kidney stones	2020

References

1. Takayama M, et al. Restriction endonuclease analysis of viral DNA from a patient with bilateral herpes zoster lesions. J Infect Dis. 1988;157:392.
2. Yoo KH, et al. Herpes zoster duplex bilateralis in a patient with breast cancer. Cancer Res Treat. 2009;41(1):50–2.
3. Vijay A, et al. Herpes zoster duplex bilateralis in immuno-competent patients: report of two cases. J Clin Diagn Res. 2015;9(12):WR01-3.

Chapter 17
Asymptomatic Erythematous Discoloration

Katerina Damevska and Stefana Damevska

A 52 years old, Caucasian man presented with more than 10 years history of skin lesions on the upper chest, neck, and lateral aspects of the face (Figs. 17.1, 17.2, and 17.3). The patient, Fitzpatrick skin type III, had a history of chronic sun exposure,

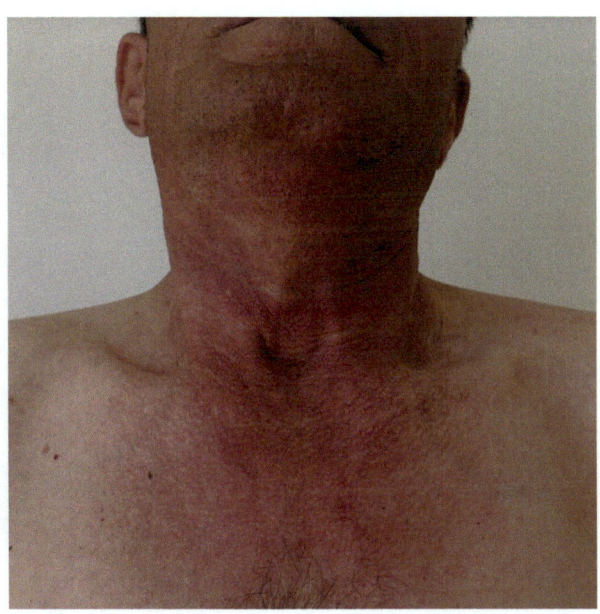

Fig. 17.1 Erythematous reticular patches with telangiectasias on the neck, lateral cheeks, and a V-shaped distribution on the upper chest. Notice sparing of the submental area shaded by the chin. Front view

K. Damevska (✉)
University Clinic for Dermatology, Faculty of Medicine, Ss Cyril and Methodius University, Skopje, Macedonia

S. Damevska
Department of Dermatology, Acibadem City Clinic Tokuda Hospital, Sofia, Bulgaria

T. M. Lotti et al. (eds.), *Clinical Cases in Facial Erythema*, Clinical Cases in Dermatology, https://doi.org/10.1007/978-3-031-05996-4_17

Fig. 17.2 Lateral left view

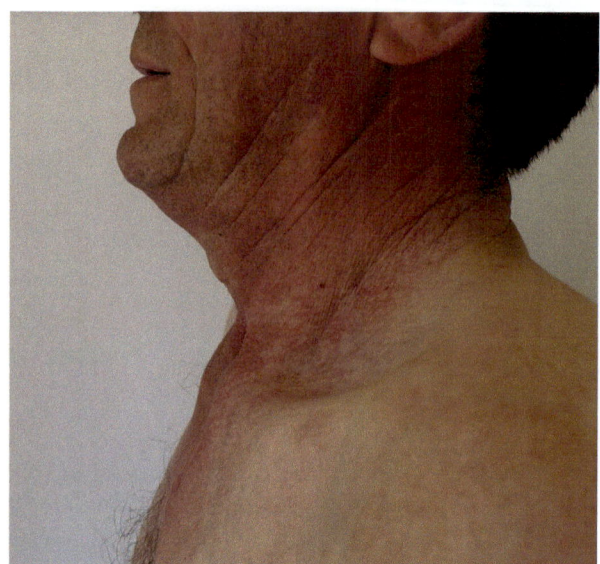

Fig. 17.3 Lateral right view

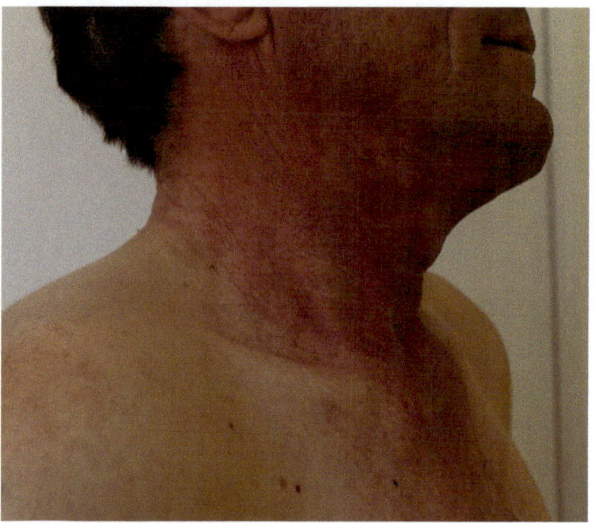

without adequate use of sunscreen protection. He was otherwise a healthy man with no history of medications, long-term use of cosmetics, fragrances, or other topical products for the skin. There was no history of photosensitivity and no personal or family history of autoimmune or thyroid disease. The patient was initially treated with topical corticosteroids and tacrolimus, without improvement.

Physical examination revealed erythematous reticular patches with superficial atrophy and occasional hyperpigmentation located in sun-exposed areas of the neck (Figs. 17.1, 17.2, and 17.3).

Based on the Case Description and the Photograph, What Is Your Diagnosis?

1. Melasma
2. Poikiloderma of Civatte
3. Acanthosis nigricans
4. Erythema dyschromicum perstans
5. Pigmented contact dermatitis (Riehl's melanosis)
6. Erythromelanosis follicularis faciei et colli

Diagnosis

Poikiloderma of Civatte.

Discussion

Poikiloderma is a combination of linear telangiectasia, mottled hyperpigmentation or depigmentation, and superficial atrophy in a reticular pattern. Poikiloderma of Civatte, also known as cervical idiopathic poikiloderma, is a benign dermatosis first described in 1923 by the French dermatologist Achilles Civatte [1].

Data concerning the prevalence of the disease is lacking. In Greece, the incidence is estimated to be 1.4% among dermatologic patients. In Civatte's original description, it was emphasized that the condition affected menopausal women. In males, the condition may be under-reported because many do not seek medical advice. Lighter skin phototypes (I–III) are more commonly affected and those engaged in outdoor occupation [1].

The condition is characterized by a reticulate pattern of pigmentation with associated telangiectasia. It usually starts from the V of the neck and spreads gradually [1]. The condition is generally asymptomatic, but rarely patients may feel itching and burning sensations. The pigmentation is reddish to brown, with symmetrical distribution, affecting the lateral cheeks, neck, and upper third of the chest. The preauricular and parotid regions are frequently involved. Sparing of the anatomically shaded areas of the neck is highly characteristic [2]. Based on the predominating clinical feature, poikiloderma of Civatte has been classified into erythemato-telangiectatic, pigmented, and mixed type. The erythemato-telangiectatic type appears to be the most common clinical type. Recognition of the clinical type is essential for selecting the most appropriate and effective treatment [1].

Genetic predisposition, cumulative exposure to UV radiation, hormonal changes associated with menopause, and contact sensitization, mostly to perfume ingredients, have all been incriminated in its obscure aetiopathogenesis [3]. Histopathological findings include solar elastosis in the upper dermis, vasodilation, perivascular edema, hyperkeratosis, epidermal atrophy, hydropic degeneration of basal cells, dermal melanophages, and sparse lymphocytic infiltrate [4, 5].

Conditions to be considered in the differential diagnosis of poikiloderma of Civatte include congenital and acquired poikilodermas and other causes of reticulate pigmentation of the face and neck.

Erythromelanosis follicularis faciei et colli is a rare dermatosis of unknown aetiopathogenesis, described by Kitamura in 1960. It is characterized by a triad consisting of well-demarcated erythema, hyperpigmentation, and follicular papules. The disease usually starts symmetrically in the preauricular area and spreads onto temples and lateral aspects of the neck. The disease primarily affects darker-skinned young men. It affects patients of all ethnic groups, but it is predominantly seen in Asian or Middle Eastern men [6].

Riehl's melanosis occurs as a result of phototoxic or photoallergic reactions. It has been associated with many cosmetic compounds, typically bergamot oil. Spotted brown pigmentation predominates, with minimal or absent telangiectasia and smaller follicular papules. It also affects dark-skinned patients, and the face is more commonly involved than in poikiloderma of Civatte. Discontinuation of offending cosmetics results in a dramatic improvement [1].

Similar changes on the neck may be seen in the skin that has been treated previously with radiotherapy. Other conditions that should be included in the differential diagnosis are genetic skin conditions such as Rothmund-Thomson syndrome and Bloom syndrome. Connective tissue diseases (such as dermatomyositis, lupus erythematosus, and mycosis fungoides) should also be considered.

Other conditions to be considered include chronic graft-versus-host disease, berloque dermatitis, and friction melanosis [1].

Following a thorough clinical assessment, treatment decisions should be made based on the proportion of pigmented and vascular components in individual patients.

The treatments for poikiloderma of Civatte include hydroquinones, electrocoagulation, cryotherapy, chemical peels, pulsed dye laser, and argon lasers. They are relatively inefficient or inconvenient and may cause hypopigmentation to the surrounding skin [7]. Depigmenting agents, such as topical hydroquinone 2–4%, topical azelaic acid 15–20%, or kojic acid, may be useful as adjuvant therapy for the pigmented type. Laser and light-based therapies are currently state-of-the-art for the treatment of poikiloderma of Civatte. Adverse effects, such as scarring with irregular hypopigmentation, postinflammatory hyperpigmentation, posttreatment purpura, mottled appearance, crusting, and erythema, have been reported [1].

Our patient was satisfied with the explanation of the benign nature of the condition and did not require any further treatment.

Key Points
- Poikiloderma of Civatte is a benign condition associated with chronic sun exposure.
- The course is slowly progressive and irreversible.
- It is more common in fair-skinned adults, especially perimenopausal females.
- Sparing of the anatomically shaded areas of the neck is highly characteristic.
- Sun protection is recommended. The treatments are relatively ineffective, inefficient, or inconvenient.

References

1. Katoulis A, Rigopoulos D, Tzima K, Stavrianeas NG. Poikiloderma of Civatte: a review. Expert Rev Dermatol. 2012;7(4):377–82.
2. Katoulis AC, Stavrianeas NG, Georgala S, Katsarou-Katsari A, Koumantaki-Mathioudaki E, Antoniou C, Stratigos JD. Familial cases of poikiloderma of Civatte: genetic implications in its pathogenesis? Clin Exp Dermatol. 1999;24(5):385–7.
3. Katoulis AC, Stavrianeas NG, Katsarou A, Antoniou C, Georgala S, Rigopoulos D, Koumantaki E, Avgerinou G, Katsambas AD. Evaluation of the role of contact sensitization and photosensitivity in the pathogenesis of poikiloderma of Civatte. Br J Dermatol. 2002;147(3):493–7.
4. Katoulis AC, Stavrianeas NG, Georgala S, et al. Poikiloderma of Civatte: a clinical and epidemiological study. J Eur Acad Dermatol Venereol. 2005;19(4):444–8. https://doi.org/10.1111/j.1468-3083.2005.01213.x.
5. Katoulis AC, Stavrianeas NG, Panayiotides JG, Bozi E, Vamvasakis E, Kalogeromitros D, Georgala S. Poikiloderma of Civatte: a histopathological and ultrastructural study. Dermatology. 2007;214(2):177–82.
6. Griffiths CEM, Barker J, Chalmers R, Bleiker T, Chalmers R, Creamer D. Rook's textbook of dermatology. 9th ed. New York: John Wiley & Sons; 2016.
7. Meijs MM, Blok FA, de Rie MA. Treatment of poikiloderma of Civatte with the pulsed dye laser: a series of patients with severe depigmentation. J Eur Acad Dermatol Venereol. 2006;20(10):1248–51.

Chapter 18
Bilateral Periorbital Erythema

Hadir Shakshouk and Julia S. Lehman

Clinical History

A 56 year-old man, with a known history of acute myeloid leukemia (AML), presented with bilateral periorbital erythema and edema of 2 days' duration. He recently developed relapse of AML, for which he received a course of high-dose cytarabine. Clinical examination revealed bilateral periorbital erythema and edema (Fig. 18.1). No other cutaneous lesions were noted on physical examination. He denied any major trauma. The rash was neither painful nor itchy.

Fig. 18.1 Periorbital erythema and edema around both eyes

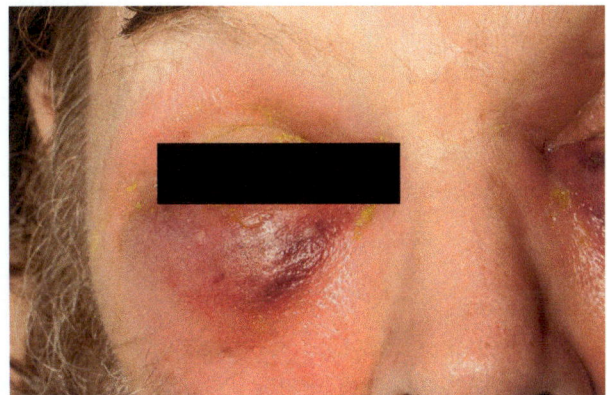

H. Shakshouk · J. S. Lehman (✉)
Department of Dermatology, Mayo Clinic, Rochester, MN, USA
e-mail: shakshouk.hadir@mayo.edu; lehman.julia@mayo.edu

T. M. Lotti et al. (eds.), *Clinical Cases in Facial Erythema*, Clinical Cases in Dermatology, https://doi.org/10.1007/978-3-031-05996-4_18

Fig. 18.2 Skin biopsy
showing neutrophilic
infiltrate surrounding the
eccrine glands (H&E,
original magnification ×20)

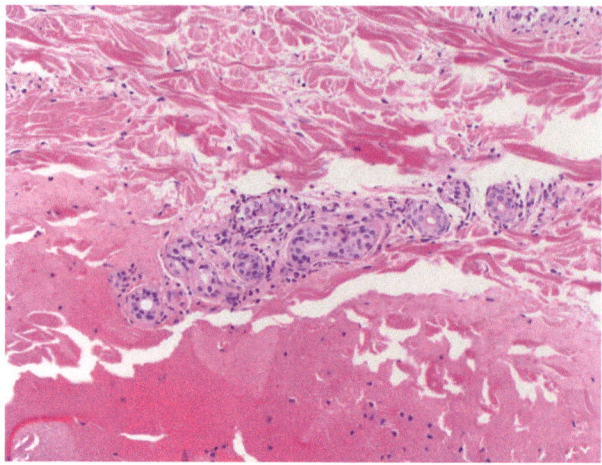

Based on the case description and the clinical photograph, **what is your diagnosis**?

1. Amyloidosis
2. Facial cellulitis
3. Necrobiotic xanthogranuloma
4. Neutrophilic eccrine hidradenitis

A skin biopsy was obtained. Histopathological examination revealed neutrophilic infiltrate present in the dermis, particularly surrounding the eccrine coils (Fig. 18.2).

Diagnosis

Neutrophilic eccrine hidradenitis induced by cytarabine.

Discussion

Neutrophilic eccrine hidradenitis (NEH) is a rare disorder reported in the setting of chemotherapy in patients with AML. Among the most commonly implicated drugs is cytarabine [1]. A wide range of drugs have also been associated with NEH including: BRAF inhibitors dabrafenib and vemurafenib [2], TNF-alpha inhibitors [3], azathioprine [4] and antiretroviral therapy. Infection with human immunodeficiency virus and various hematological and solid malignancies have also been associated [5].

NEH manifests clinically with diverse skin lesions. Erythematous papules and plaques are among the commonest features. Lesions can be asymptomatic or painful. While the trunk is a frequently involved location, involvement of the face and extremities has also been described. Lesions usually appear 10 days after initiation of chemotherapy [1]. The definite diagnosis is made by histopathological examination [5]. Typically, skin biopsy shows abundant neutrophils infiltrating the eccrine gland secretory coils with epithelial necrosis [1]. Other features previously described include: diffuse or perivascular neutrophilic infiltrate and spongiosis [1]. The exact pathogenesis remains unknown. However, it is widely thought to be a result of drug-induced cytotoxic effect on the eccrine glands [5].

Our patient has a relatively uncommon presentation, as lesions of NEH were exclusively periorbital. Although the diagnosis was confirmed by history and skin biopsy, other entities in the differential diagnosis that should be excluded include facial cellulitis [6]. Cellulitis is classically painful and lesions are more erythematous and poorly defined, unlike NEH which has lesions that tend to be more violaceous and well-ircumscribed [7].

NEH is a self-limiting disorder, which usually resolves after chemotherapy cessation. Treatment with the use of topical corticosteroids is optional [5]. Dapsone has been reported to prevent recurrence in some cases [1].

Key Points
- Neutrophilic eccrine hidradenitis is a rare disease induced by chemotherapeutic agents such as cytarabine.
- Diagnosis is made by history and skin biopsy showing neutrophilic infiltration involving eccrine glands.

References

1. Bachmeyer C, Aractingi S. Neutrophilic eccrine hidradenitis. Clin Dermatol. 2000;18:319–30. https://doi.org/10.1016/S0738-081X(99)00123-6.
2. Herms F, Franck N, Kramkimel N, Fichel F, Delaval L, Laurent-Roussel S, et al. Neutrophilic eccrine hidradenitis in two patients treated with BRAF inhibitors: a new cutaneous adverse event. Br J Dermatol. 2017;176:1645–8. https://doi.org/10.1111/bjd.15259.
3. Hawryluk EB, Linskey KR, Duncan LM, Nazarian RM. Broad range of adverse cutaneous eruptions in patients on TNF-alpha antagonists. J Cutan Pathol. 2012;39:481–92. https://doi.org/10.1111/j.1600-0560.2012.01894.x.
4. García-Martín P, Sánchez-Pérez J, Fraga J, García-Diez A. Neutrophilic eccrine hidradenitis in a patient with Crohn's disease and azathioprine hypersensitivity syndrome. J Eur Acad Dermatol Venereol. 2014;28:1830–2. https://doi.org/10.1111/jdv.12380.
5. Nelson CA, Stephen S, Ashchyan HJ, James WD, Micheletti RG, Rosenbach M. Neutrophilic dermatoses. J Am Acad Dermatol. 2018;79:987–1006. https://doi.org/10.1016/j.jaad.2017.11.064.
6. Srivastava M, Scharf S, Meehan SA, Polsky D. Neutrophilic eccrine hidradenitis masquerading as facial cellulitis. J Am Acad Dermatol. 2007;56:693–6. https://doi.org/10.1016/j.jaad.2006.07.032.
7. Copaescu A-M, Castilloux J-F, Chababi-Atallah M, Sinave C, Bertrand J. A classic clinical case: neutrophilic eccrine hidradenitis. Case Rep Dermatol. 2013;5:340–6. https://doi.org/10.1159/000356229.

Chapter 19
Cutaneous Angiosarcoma on Scalp and Face in an Elderly Patient

Jin-Fa Dou, Jian-Bo Wang, Hui Li, Yu-Ping Wang, and Shou-Min Zhang

A 70-year-old male presented with the dark red plaques for 10 years, nodules and ulcers for 1 year on the scalp and facial ecchymosis for 2 months (Fig. 19.1).

Red patches occurred on the top of the head 10 years ago, without any symptoms. There were some nodules scattering around the red patches 1 year ago, followed by ulceration. He was treated as an "hemangioma" with the injection of pingyangmycin in the local hospital. After more than 20 days of injection, the red nodules became dry and crusted off. But the nodules reappeared 2 months ago and

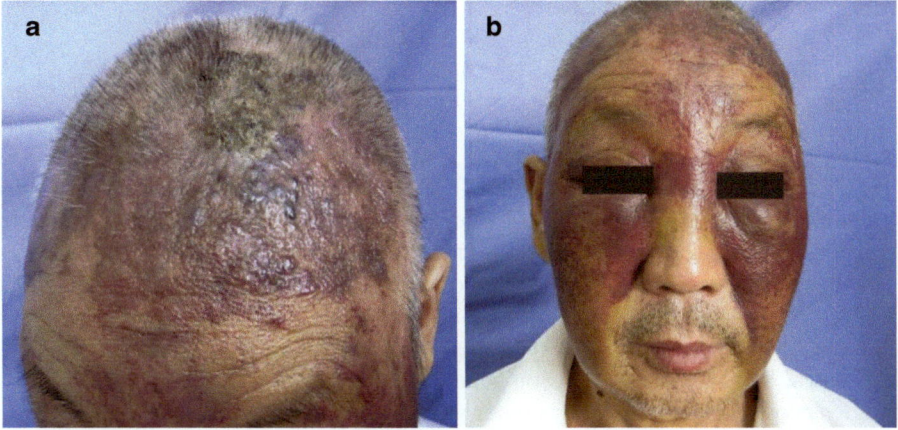

Fig. 19.1 Clinical manifestation of the patient. (**a**) Nodules and ulcers on the scalp; (**b**) purple ecchymosis on the face

J.-F. Dou · J.-B. Wang · H. Li · Y.-P. Wang · S.-M. Zhang (✉)
Department of Dermatology, Henan Provincial People's Hospital, People's Hospital of Zhengzhou University, People's Hospital of Henan University, Zhengzhou, China

pingyangmycin was given again. It is regrettable that 2 h after the injection, her face appeared bright red patches accompanied by edema of both eyelids, and erythema area gradually enlarged and turned purple-red.

Based on the Case Description and the Photograph, What Is Your Diagnosis?

1. Nevus flammeus
2. Kaposi's Sarcoma
3. Cutaneous angiosarcoma

Histological examination of a skin lesion biopsy revealed the signs for a large number of newly formed vascular cavities and heteromorphic mitosis. Immunostaining for both CD34 and CD31 were positive.

Diagnosis

Cutaneous angiosarcoma.

Discussion

Cutaneous angiosarcoma (cAS) derived from vascular endothelial cells is a rare and highly aggressive malignant neoplasm [1]. Multiple aetiological factors may play a role in cAS, including lymphostasis, radiation and chronic sun exposure. cAS is a genetically heterogeneous tumors based on the cancer genomic studies. Mutations in several pathways are responsible for cAS, such as TP53, PTPRB, PLCG1, CDKN2A and MYC, in which, the mutation in the TP53 gene, responsible for tumour suppressor protein p53 synthesis, is one of the most common mutations in AS cases. Recently, a novel fusion gene, NUP160-SCL43A3, was identified in an angiosarcoma cell line and may confer growth advantage to the cells [2].

cAS generally affects the face, scalp and neck of the elders with high frequency in men than women. cAS manifests a haematoma-like lesion with no symptoms initially, and develops into nodule, papule, plaque and exophytic tumour on the surface of progressing lesions. AS is classified into primary AS and secondary AS. Secondary AS is usually related to a history of radiation therapy and chronic lymphedema. The radiation-associated angiosarcoma (RAAS) is the most complication of radiation treatment with the latency period at 2–30 years with a median of 5 years [3, 4]. The development of AS in the setting of chronic lymphoedema was termed as Stewart–Treves syndrome [5]. Prognosis of cAS is poor with medial survival about 3.4–5 years because of a high rate of local recurrence and tendency to metastasis [6].

Nevus flammeus common affect infants, and present pink patch on the skin, mostly in the face or the limb. As the child gets older, the discoloration will darken to a purple or deep red color. Histopathological examination shows mature endothelial cells without endothelial cell proliferation.

Kaposi's Sarcoma (KS) typically appear as painless purplish spots or patches on the legs, feet or face. KS is related to the infection with human herpesvirus-8 (HHV-8) under the condition of immune deficiency, including HIV infection and drugs taken after an organ transplant, or another disease. Histopathology manifests a malignant tumor of hemorrhagic vascular endothelial cells, with proliferation of slit-like blood vessels, endothelial cells protruding into the lumen and extravasation of erythrocytes. Nuclear atypia is usually less prominent in KS, unlike in cAS. Nuclear expression of HHV-8 by immunohistochemistry is seen in KS but not AS.

Based on the patient's medical history, clinical manifestation and histopathological examination and immunohistochemistry result, the diagnosis of AS was made. Of note, AS has a very poor prognosis due to the high rate of involved lymph nodes and distant metastasis, therefore, early and proper diagnosis and treatment are necessary. Early surgery and extensive excision is the key to reducing mortality, and the combination of surgery and radiation/chemotherapy is the mainstay of treatment for AS.

Key Points
- Cutaneous angiosarcoma (cAS) is a rare malignant neoplasm with a haematoma-like lesion.
- Histopathological examination and immunohistochemistry are necessary in the differential diagnosis of cAS and other vascular proliferative disease.

References

1. Ishida Y, et al. Cutaneous angiosarcoma: update on biology and latest treatment. Curr Opin Oncol. 2018;30(2):107–12.
2. Shimozono N, et al. NUP160-SLC43A3 is a novel recurrent fusion oncogene in angiosarcoma. Cancer Res. 2015;75(21):4458–65.
3. Lindford A, et al. Surgical management of radiation-associated cutaneous breast angiosarcoma. J Plast Reconstr Aesthet Surg. 2011;64(8):1036–42.
4. Mery CM, et al. Secondary sarcomas after radiotherapy for breast cancer: sustained risk and poor survival. Cancer. 2009;115(18):4055–63.
5. Sasajima J, et al. Pancreatic metastasis of angiosarcoma (Stewart-Treves syndrome) diagnosed using endoscopic ultrasound-guided fine needle aspiration: a case report. Medicine. 2016;95(33):e4316.
6. Dettenborn T, et al. Prognostic features in angiosarcoma of the head and neck: a retrospective monocenter study. J Craniomaxillofac Surg. 2014;42(8):1623–8.

Chapter 20
Disseminated Vesicular Lesions in an Immunocompetent Individual

Shashank Bhargava and George Kroumpouzos

A 43-year-old male patient presented to dermatology with complaints of stabbing pain and a rash consisting of multiple grouped fluid-filled lesions on the right side of the chest for 3 days. A day before the grouped lesions appeared, discrete vesicular lesions developed over the face, neck, back and chest. Skin examination showed grouped tense vesicles and a few bullae on an erythematous base involving T4–T5 dermatome (Fig. 20.1). Lesions were associated with severe pain and burning sensation. Also, numerous discrete papulovesicles were noted on the face, neck, and back (Fig. 20.2). Patient was afebrile, and there was no history of weight loss or malignancy. He was not on any immunosuppressive medications. Ultrasonograph of the abdomen was normal. Serum glucose and HBA1C were within normal limits. Human immunodeficiency virus (HIV) testing was negative. Cultures (blood, urine, cerebrospinal fluid) were negative. Tumor markers and anti-VZV IgM antibody tests were also negative. A Tzanck smear revealed multinucleated giant cells (Fig. 20.3).

S. Bhargava
Department of Dermatology, R.D. Gardi Medical College, Ujjain, India

G. Kroumpouzos (✉)
Department of Dermatology, Alpert Medical School of Brown University, Providence, RI, USA

GK Dermatology, PC, South Weymouth, MA, USA
e-mail: gk@gkderm.com

© The Author(s), under exclusive license to Springer Nature Switzerland AG 2022
T. M. Lotti et al. (eds.), *Clinical Cases in Facial Erythema*, Clinical Cases in Dermatology, https://doi.org/10.1007/978-3-031-05996-4_20

Fig. 20.1 Grouped minute
blisters on an erythematous
base are noted on the right
chest; the lesions extend
onto the right axilla

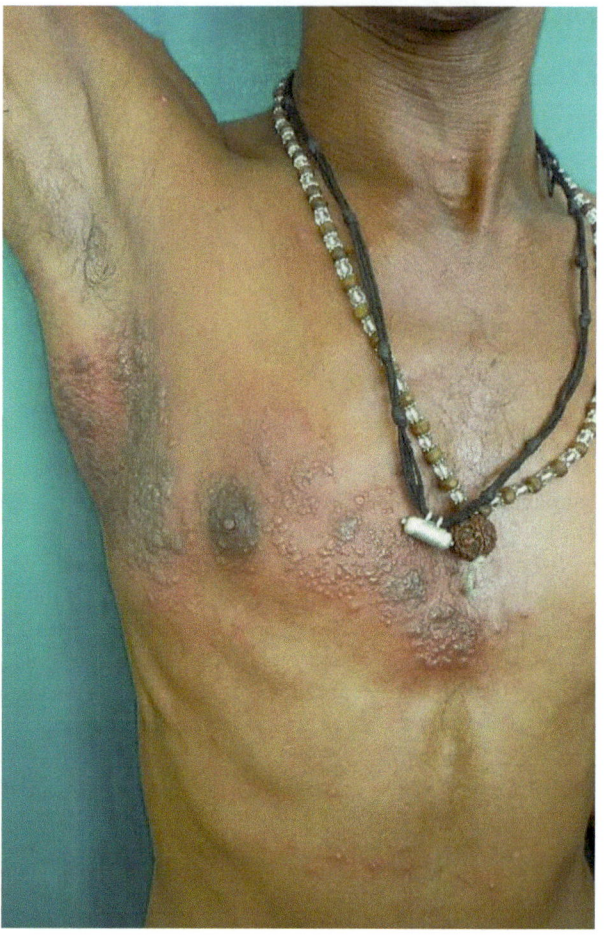

Based on the Case Description and Photographs, What Is Your Diagnosis?

- Eczema herpeticum
- Primary varicella infection
- Disseminated herpes zoster
- Paedrous dermatitis with *id* reaction
- Allergic contact dermatitis

Diagnosis

Disseminated herpes zoster. The diagnosis is supported by the clinical findings, i.e., >20 vesicles away from the primary involved dermatome, and a positive Tzanck smear.

Fig. 20.2 Discrete pink to erythematous papulovesicles and crusts on the face

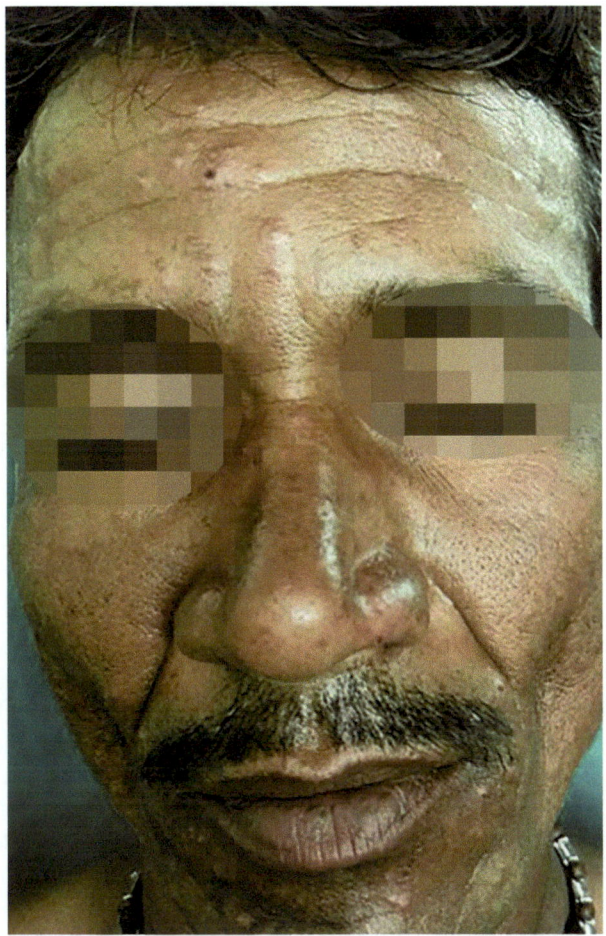

Discussion

Varicella-zoster virus (VZV) causes varicella (also called chickenpox), herpes zoster (also called shingles), and rarely, a severe disseminated disease that can manifest with a generalized eruption, encephalitis, hepatitis, and pneumonitis. Disseminated disease affects mainly immunocompromised patients [1]. The reactivation of VZV is related to a decrease in VZV-specific T-cell immunity. With increasing age, the cell-mediated immunity decreases, which increases the incidence of herpes zoster and postherpetic neuralgia [2]. A disseminated herpes zoster infection can be diagnosed when 20 or more blisters develop outside the area of primary and adjacent dermatomes within a week of development dermatomal involvement and symptoms typical of herpes zoster infection [3]. Dissemination of herpes zoster infection is uncommon. It has been reported predominantly in immunocompromised elderly people, patients with HIV or hematologic malignancies, or those on chemotherapy [4, 5].

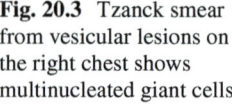

Fig. 20.3 Tzanck smear
from vesicular lesions on
the right chest shows
multinucleated giant cells

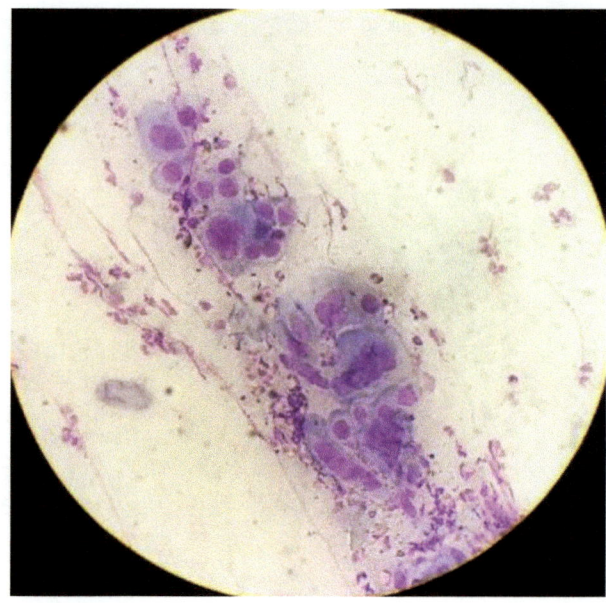

Here, we describe a rare case of disseminated herpes zoster in an immunocompetent young patient. This case is unusual in that clinical differentiation from varicella was challenging while the laboratory test findings (negative anti-VZV IgM) were consistent with herpes zoster. VZV IgM is extremely rare during VZV reactivation, and even if positive, the titers are not high [3]. The dermatomal distribution of clustered truncal lesions (T4–T5) favors herpes zoster in our case. Our patient was started on oral valacyclovir and analgesics. Symptoms resolved by the fourth day, and no new skin lesions developed after the third day of treatment. To enhance prompt diagnosis and initiation of therapy, clinicians should be aware of atypical presentations of VZV infection.

Key Points
- A disseminated herpes zoster infection can be diagnosed when 20 or more blisters develop systemically within a week of showing skin symptoms found in typical herpes zoster infections.
- Extensive cutaneous dissemination has been reported in immune-compromised patients, such as those who suffer from HIV infections, cancer, chemotherapy, and corticosteroid therapy patients.
- Disseminated herpes zoster in a young immunocompetent individual is rare and should be evaluated with keen observation because the discrete lesions are the first to appear.

References

1. Brown TJ, McCrary M, Tyring SK. Varicella-zoster virus (herpes 3). J Am Acad Dermatol. 2002;47:972–97.
2. Arvin A. Aging, immunity, and the varicella-zoster virus. N Engl J Med. 2005;352:2266–7.
3. Gupta S, Jain A, Gardiner C, Tyring SK. A rare case of disseminated cutaneous zoster in an immunocompetent patient. BMC Fam Pract. 2005;6:50.
4. Mishra AK, Sahu KK, James A. Disseminated herpes zoster following treatment with benralizumab. Clin Respir J. 2019;13:189–91.
5. Shum D, Arenas CG. Disseminated herpes zoster. J Am Osteopath Assoc. 2015;115:175.

Chapter 21
Erythematous Papular Lesions of the Face

Erdal Polat, Muazzez Cigdem Oba, and Zekayi Kutlubay

Case

Fifty-four year-old female, with no medical antecedents, presented to our clinic with a four-year history of recurrent erythema and rash on the cheeks. She reported associated pruritus and stinging sensation. On dermatologic examination, the patient had numerous papules and pustules on an erythematous base on the cheeks (Fig. 21.1). She was previously diagnosed as papulopustular rosacea. Her past treatments included topical and systemic antibiotics and systemic isotretinoin, which were ineffective. She denied topical steroid use.

Microbiological examination was performed using standardized superficial skin biopsy. For this purpose, a clean glass slide covered with cyanoacrylate glue was put on the lesion, and removed after 1 min, which allowed the collection follicular components. Light microscopic examination of 1 cm^2 of the slide revealed 7 *Demodex folliculorum* mites (Fig. 21.2).

Permethrin 5% cream twice daily was prescribed. Full clearance of the lesion was achieved as early as at 2 weeks (Fig. 21.3).

E. Polat
İstanbul University-Cerrahpaşa, Cerrahpaşa Medical Faculty, Department of Microbiology, İstanbul, Turkey

M. C. Oba
Health Sciences University, Sancaktepe Şehit Prof. Dr. İlhan Varank Research and Training Hospital, Department of Dermatology, İstanbul, Turkey
e-mail: muazzez.oba@istanbul.edu.tr

Z. Kutlubay (✉)
İstanbul University-Cerrahpaşa, Cerrahpaşa Medical Faculty, Department of Dermatology, İstanbul, Turkey

T. M. Lotti et al. (eds.), *Clinical Cases in Facial Erythema*, Clinical Cases in Dermatology, https://doi.org/10.1007/978-3-031-05996-4_21

Fig. 21.1 Papules and pustules on an erythematous base on the left cheek

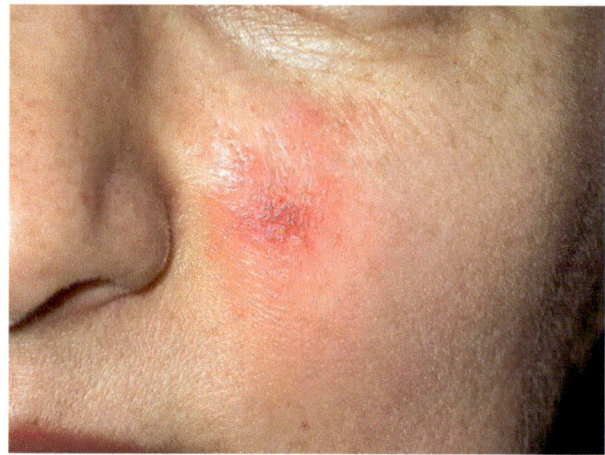

Fig. 21.2 *Demodex folliculorum* mites on light microscopic examination

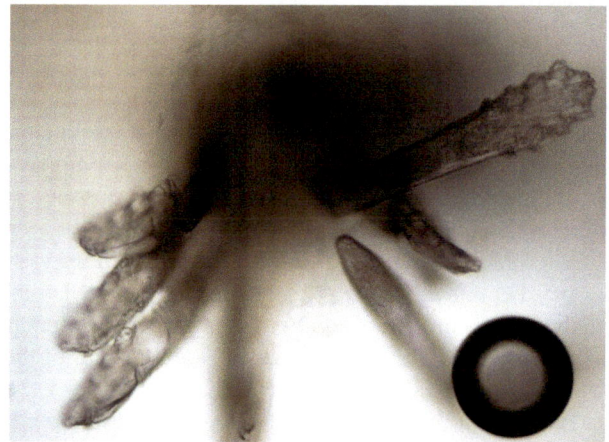

Fig. 21.3 Complete clearance of the lesion after topical permethrin therapy

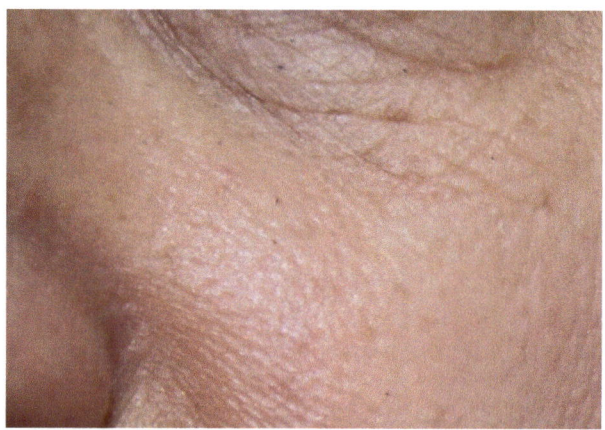

Based on the case description and the findings, what is your diagnosis?

• Acne vulgaris
• Gram negative folliculitis
• Allergic contact dermatitis

Diagnosis

Rosacea with *Demodex* mite infestation.

Discussion

Rosacea is a chronic skin disease of the central face, characterized by transient or persistent erythema, telangiectasia, papules, pustules, ocular and pyhmatous lesions. Four subtypes of the disease, namely, erythematotelangiectatic, papulopustular, phymatous, ocular; and one variant, granulomatous rosacea have been defined. Pathophysiology of the disease is unclear [1]. However, *Demodex* mites have been shown to play a pathogenic role in erythemato-telangiectatic rosacea (ETR) and papulopustular rosacea (PPR). Patients with ETR and PPR have a significantly higher prevalence and density of *Demodex* mite infestation. *Demodex* infestation or demodicosis is defined as *Demodex* density of five or more mites per cm^2 and association with pathogenic activity [2]. Rosacea like demodicosis and PPR can be considered as two phenotypes of the same disease [3]. In addition, patients presenting with lesions resembling PPR should be questioned about topical steroid use. The latter can lead to PPR like eruption that typically involves perioral region sparing vermillion border [4].

Topical metronidazole, azelaic acid and topical ivermectin are included in the first line treatment options of mild-to-moderate PPR. Topical ivermectin has dual mechanism of action by being both anti-inflammatory and acaricidal against *Demodex* mites [5]. Another antiparasitic agent, topical permethrin also effectively reduces inflammatory lesions and Demodex density [6]. Combination of topical therapies and systemic drug treatments (e.g. tetracyclines or isotretinoin) is recommended for moderate-to-severe PPR [5].

Acne vulgaris presents with inflammatory papules and pustules and perilesional erythema, similar to PPR. However, several clues help in their differential diagnosis [7]. Rosacea typically affects patients between 30 and 50 years of age, whereas acne tends to affect patients at a younger age [5, 7]. Burning and stinging that are common symptoms of rosacea, are not reported in acne. Clinically, comedones, scarring and involvement of areas other then the face such as chest and back are observed in acne [4, 7]. Lastly, demodicosis is significantly more associated with rosacea than acne [2].

Gram negative folliculitis presents with persistent papulopustular lesions. It occurs as a result of prolonged oral antibiotic therapy, which alters normal skin flora. Culture of the pustules reveals Gram negative pathogens such as Escherichia coli, Klebsiella, Enterobacter and Proteus species [4].

Allergic contact dermatitis of the face occurs due to facial skin care products, cosmetics and sometimes as a result of topical therapies [7]. It can result in erythema, papules and pustules along with burning and stinging [8]. A careful history and patch testing is useful for diagnosis of allergic contact dermatitis [7].

Key Points
- Patients presenting with lesions resembling papulopustular rosacea should be questioned about topical steroid use.
- *Demodex* mites have been shown to play a pathogenic role in erythematotelangiectatic rosacea and papulopustular rosacea.
- Standardized superficial skin biopsy is a practical method to determine *Demodex* density.
- Antiparasitic agents such as ivermectin and permethrin should be considered in the treatment of rosacea patients with demodicosis.

References

1. Wilkin J, Dahl M, Detmar M, Drake L, Feinstein A, Odom R, et al. Standard classification of rosacea: report of the National Rosacea Society expert committee on the classification and staging of rosacea. J Am Acad Dermatol. 2002;46:584–7.
2. Chang YS, Huang YC. Role of demodex mite infestation in rosacea: a systematic review and meta-analysis. J Am Acad Dermatol. 2017;77:441–7.
3. Forton FMN, De Maertelaer V. Papulopustular rosacea and rosacea-like demodicosis: two phenotypes of the same disease? J Eur Acad Dermatol Venereol. 2018;32(6):1011–6.
4. Johnson SM, Berg A, Barr C. Recognizing Rosacea: Tips on Differential Diagnosis. J Drugs Dermatol. 2019;18:888–94.
5. Ebbelaar CCF, Venema AW, Van Dijk MR. Topical ivermectin in the treatment of papulopustular rosacea: a systematic review of evidence and clinical guideline recommendations. Dermatol Ther (Heidelb). 2018;8:379–87.
6. Raoufinejad K, Mansouri P, Rajabi M, Naraghi Z, Jebraeili R. Efficacy and safety of permethrin 5% topical gel vs. placebo for rosacea: a double-blind randomized controlled clinical trial. J Eur Acad Dermatol Venereol. 2016;30:2105–17.
7. Dessinioti C, Antoniou C. The "red face": not always rosacea. Clin Dermatol. 2017;35:201–6.
8. Culp B, Scheinfeld N. Rosacea: a review. P T. 2009;34(1):38–45.

Chapter 22
Facial Erythema and Flushing in a 55-Year-Old Female

Tugba Kevser Uzuncakmak and Zekayi Kutlubay

Case

A 55-year-old female presented to the dermatology department with a 2-year history of flushing and redness on her face. Clinical examination revealed widespread erythema and extensive telangiectasias on bilateral cheeks and chin (Fig. 22.1). On dermoscopic examination polygonal vessels, superficial scales, follicular plugs, and features related to demodicosis were detected.

Her laboratory tests including complete blood counting, biochemistry, erythrocyte sedimentation rate, rheumatoid factor, complement levels, urinalysis, and serologic tests including antinuclear anticore, anti-ds DNA were normal.

Based on the case description and the photograph, what is your diagnosis?

- Lupus erythematosus
- Acne rosacea
- Dermatomyositis
- DRESS (Drug reaction with eosinophilia and systemic manifestations.)

Diagnosis

Acne rosacea.

T. K. Uzuncakmak (✉) · Z. Kutlubay
Istanbul University-Cerrahpasa, Cerrahpasa Medical Faculty, Department of Dermatology, Fatih, Istanbul, Turkey

© The Author(s), under exclusive license to Springer Nature Switzerland AG 2022
T. M. Lotti et al. (eds.), *Clinical Cases in Facial Erythema*, Clinical Cases in Dermatology, https://doi.org/10.1007/978-3-031-05996-4_22

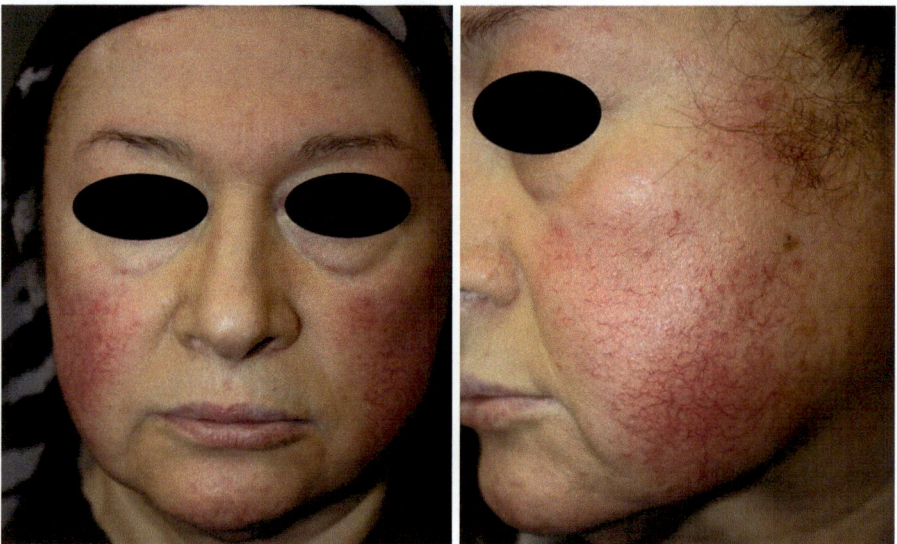

Fig. 22.1 Widespread erythema and extensive telangiectasias on bilateral cheeks and chin

Discussion

Acne rosacea is a common, chronic, inflammatory, and multifactorial dermatosis that is mainly affecting the centrofacial region [1]. It is estimated to affect 2–20% f the population worldwide and it has a complex etiopathogenesis, including immunological dysregulation, genetic predisposition, and neurogenic inflammation [2]. It is more common in female, lighter skin phototypes, between the ages of 30–60. It is characterized by symptoms of flushing and facial erythema, edema, burning and stinging senses, telangiectasia, the coarseness of skin, and in the papulopustular form an inflammatory papulopustular eruption resembling acne vulgaris [3]. Comedones are usually absent in clinical examination and this finding may be helpful in the differential diagnosis from classical acne. Lesions are usually localized on the nose, cheeks, and forehead. Rosacea was classified into four main subtypes by The National Rosacea Society according to the specific clinical signs and symptoms including erythematotelangiectatic type, papulopustular type, phymatous and ocular subtype [1]. These subtypes may appear individually or may progress to another subtype eventually. Histologically, in nonpustular lesions, a nonspecific perivascular and perifollicular lymphohistiocytic infiltrate, plasma cells, multinucleated cells, eosinophils and neutrophils may be detected, whereas in papulopustular lesions a more intensive granulomatous inflammation and perifollicular abscesses may be seen, and also *Demodex folliculorum* may be seen in follicles.

Treatment modalities change according to the disease subtype and severity. Topical agents may help in disease control. The most cited topical agents are topical metronidazole gel/cream, alpha-1 adrenergic receptor agonists (brimonidine tartrate

0.5% gel and oxymetazoline 1% cream), ivermectin, permethrin cream, azelaic acid gel/cream. Systemic cyclin group antibiotics, metronidazole, isotretinoin, and beta-adrenergic receptor antagonists may be effective [1]. In addition to management protocols avoiding triggering factors such as hot drinks, hot or cold temperatures, wind, caffeine, spicy foods, alcohol, exercise, topical irritant agents, and medications which may lead to flushing should be recommended [2]. Vascular lasers may be helpful in the erythematotelangiectatic type via using wavelengths allowing the selective absorption by oxyhemoglobin that leads to reduction in vessels without causing a scarring or damage to surrounding skin. Electrosurgery or the 585-nm pulsed dye laser may effective in patients who have permanent telangiectasia. However, facial erythema may not improved, or new telangiectasias may occur again over time. Cosmetic improvement can be achieved in rhinophyma patients via mechanical dermabrasion, carbon dioxide laser peeling, and surgical shave techniques.

Also, the use of daily broad-spectrum sunscreen should be recommended for all patients with rosacea.

The lupus erythematosus (LE) is a multifactorial, multisystemic connective-tissue disorder. It is related to polyclonal B-cell activation and occurs as a result of the complex interaction of immunologic, environmental, hormonal, and genetic factors [4]. The clinical findings of LE can vary from localized or limited cutaneous disease to generalized systemic disease. From the point of dermatological view LE–specific skin diseases were classified into three categories including acute cutaneous lupus erythematosus, subacute cutaneous lupus erythematosus, and chronic cutaneous lupus erythematosus. Although clinically each group has different findings, histopathologically, they usually represent similar features. In patients with acute cutaneous LE, a typical malar eruption in a butterfly pattern localized to the central portion of the face sparing the nasolabial folds and/or a more generalized maculopapular eruption representing a photosensitive dermatitis is detected. Antinuclear antibody (ANA), anti-dsDNA and complement levels are helpful in the differential diagnosis.

Dermatomyositis is an idiopathic inflammatory disease that is characterized by cutaneous findings and myopathy that may affect both children and adults [2]. The skin and muscles are the most commonly affected tissues but as a systemic disorder, it may also affect the joints; and internal organs. The sole cutaneous manifestation may be seen in 40% of individuals with dermatomyositis. The most common cutaneous findings are pruritic erythematous, scaly papules and plaques predominantly on photo-exposed surfaces, especially on the mid-face, malar erythema, poikiloderma in sun-exposed areas, the heliotrope rash that consists of a violaceous to erythematous rash along the eyelid margins, with or without periorbital edema and the Gottron papules which are flat-topped, erythematous to violaceous papules and plaques found over the dorsal aspect of hands, particularly over the knuckles [2]. Muscle enzyme levels and serologic abnormalities may be helpful in the differential diagnosis, but these antibodies were found to be positive in 30% of the patients with dermatomyositis or polymyositis. Antinuclear antibody positivity is common in patients with dermatomyositis but not necessary for diagnosis. Anti –mi-2 antibodies also have a high specificity with low sensitivity. This antibody is positive especially in patients who have acute onset disease, V neck sign, and shawl rash. Anti-Jo-1 antibodies are more common in polymyositis.

DRESS (Drug reaction with eosinophilia and systemic manifestations) syndrome, also known as drug-induced hypersensitivity syndrome, is one of the most severe cutaneous adverse reaction that can be potentially life-threatening [5]. It is more commonly reported with anticonvulsants and sulfonamides but various drugs may induce this reaction. A maculopapular cutaneous eruption accompanied by fever and lymphadenopathy is the most common clinical manifestation of DRESS syndrome. Lesions may appear 2-6 weeks following the offending agent intake. Usually, leukocytosis and abnormal liver tests are present at the time with cutaneous lesions. Cutaneous lesions are usually characterized by urticarial, maculopapular lesions, however vesicular, bullous, pustular, purpuric, targetoid lesions, or even erythroderma can be also seen. Facial edema is a characteristic of DRESS. Clinical prognosis is associated with systemic involvement, which may lead to multi-organ failure. Early diagnosis and immediate cessation of the suspected offending drug is the most important step in the management of DRESS.

Key Points
- Acne rosacea is a common, chronic, inflammatory, and multifactorial dermatosis that is mainly affecting the centrofacial region, scalp, and ocular region.
- Acne rosacea is more commonly seen in female, lighter skin phototypes, between the ages of 30-60.
- Clinically acne rosacea is characterized by symptoms of flushing and facial erythema, edema, burning and stinging senses, telangiectasia, the coarseness of skin and in the papulopustular form an inflammatory papulopustular eruption resembling acne vulgaris.
- Clinically it may mimic several inflammatory facial lesions. Dermoscopy may be helpful in the differential diagnosis.
- Topical metronidazole gel/cream, alpha-1 adrenergic receptor agonists (brimonidine tartrate 0.5% gel and oxymetazoline 1% cream), ivermectin, permethrin cream, azelaic acid gel/cream may be helpful in the local management of acne rosacea
- Systemic cyclin group antibiotics, metronidazole, isotretinoin, and beta-adrenergic receptor antagonists may be effective in persistent and patients who have extensive involvement.
- Patients should avoid triggering factors such as hot or cold temperatures, wind, hot drinks, caffeine, exercise, spicy foods, alcohol, topical products that irritate the skin, and medications that cause flushing should be recommended.
- Laser treatments may be helpful in erythematotelangiectatic type.
- In rhinophyma patients, mechanical dermabrasion, carbon dioxide laser peeling, and surgical shave techniques are more effective.
- Daily use of broad-spectrum sunscreen should be recommended for all patients with rosacea.

References

1. Oliveira CMM, Almeida LMC, Bonamigo RR, Lima CWG, Bagatin E. Consensus on the therapeutic management of rosacea - Brazilian Society of Dermatology. An Bras Dermatol. 2020;95:53–69.
2. Dessinioti C, Antoniou C. The "red face": not always rosacea. Clin Dermatol. 2017;35:201–6.
3. İkizoğlu G. Red face revisited: flushing. Clin Dermatol. 2014;32:800–8.
4. Errichetti E, Lallas A, De Marchi G, Apalla Z, Zabotti A, De Vita S, Stinco G. Dermoscopy in the differential diagnosis between malar rash of systemic lupus erythematosus and erythemato-telangiectatic rosacea: an observational study. Lupus. 2019;28:1583–8.
5. De A, Rajagopalan M, Sarda A, Das S, Biswas P. Drug reaction with eosinophilia and systemic symptoms: an update and review of recent literature. Indian J Dermatol. 2018;63:30–40.

Chapter 23
Generalised Exfoliating "Figurate Erythema": A Rare Cause

Lawrence Chukwudi Nwabudike and Alin Laurentiu Tatu

Short Clinical Case History

A 41-year old male, construction worker presented with a 4-month history of generalised itchy rash. There was no apparent exacerbation in relation to work, though he noted that it followed a period of stress from not being paid money he was owed. Patch testing suggested copper sensitivity. He had been treated with topical and systemic steroids (methylprednisolone and prednisone), topical and systemic antifungals (naftifine, terbinafine, fluconazole), as well as antihistamines (desloratadine, loratadine) with no lasting effect.

The patient's medical history was sivgnificant for a right inguinal herniorrhaphy. He smoked 30 cigarettes daily for over 20 years and drank about 660 ml of beer/day.

Examination revealed a patient with an athletic build and erthematosquamous plaques, many with annular configuration and central clearing (Figs. 23.1 and 23.2). In some cases, the active squamous margin was on the inner margins of the erythematous rings.

L. C. Nwabudike (✉)
N. Paulescu National Institute of Diabetes, Bucharest, Romania

A. L. Tatu
Faculty of Medicine and Pharmacy/Clinical Department, Dermatology, Medical and Pharmaceutical Research Unit/Competitive, Interdisciplinary Research Integrated Platform "Dunărea de Jos", ReForm-UDJG "Dunărea de Jos" University, Galati, Romania

Infectious Diseases Clinical Hospital "St. Parascheva", Dermatology, Galati, Romania

Multidisciplinary Integrated Center of Dermatological Interface Research MIC-DIR, 'Dunarea de Jos' University, Galati, Romania

T. M. Lotti et al. (eds.), *Clinical Cases in Facial Erythema*, Clinical Cases in Dermatology, https://doi.org/10.1007/978-3-031-05996-4_23

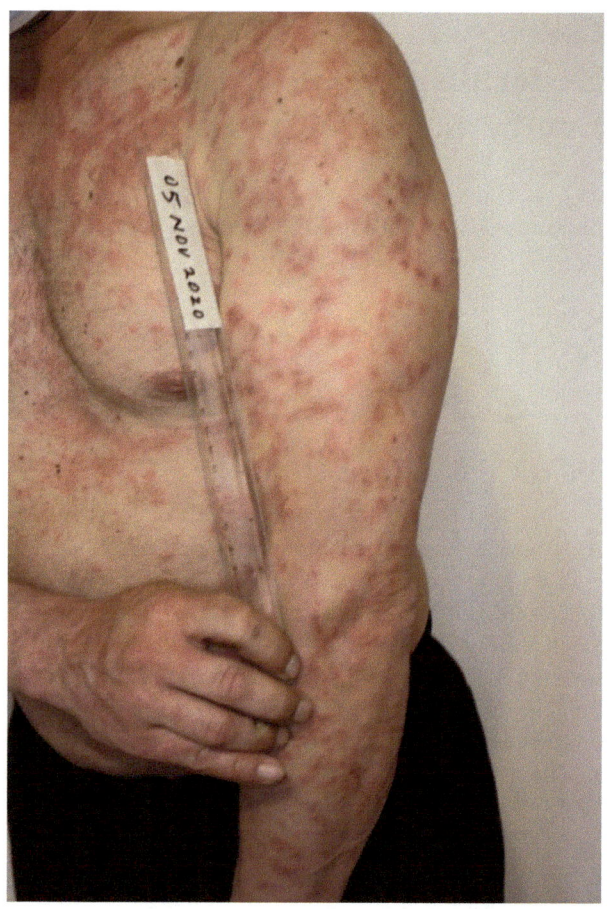

Fig. 23.1 Erythematous, annular rash, with central clearing, in a generalised distribution

What Is Your Diagnosis?

1. Erythema annulare centrifugum
2. Erythema marginatum
3. Annular psoriasis
4. Generalised eczema
5. Generalised fixed drug eruption

Diagnosis

Generalised fixed drug eruption.

Fig. 23.2 Erythematous rash with some lesions in a serpeginous distribution on right lateral thorax

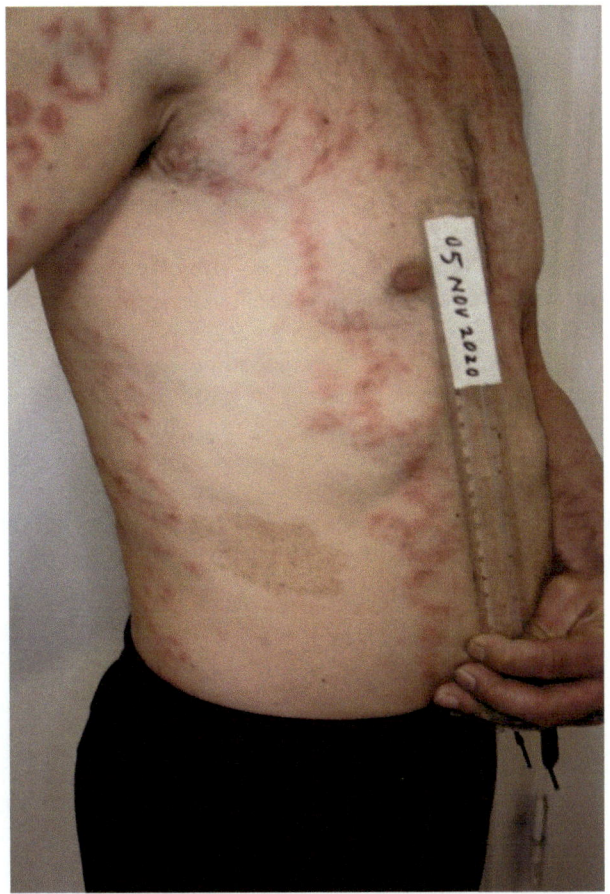

Discussion

The patient's histopathology suggested fixed drug eruption.

Fixed drug eruptions can be localised or generalised and are an allergic reaction to a drug. Sometimes, as in the present case, the offending drug may be unknown. Generalised fixed drug eruption (GFDE) is less common than localised fixed drug eruption [1]. It may be bullous or non-bullous, with the bullous variety being more common [1]. Ingested antibiotics appear to be a common cause of the non-bullous variety [1, 2], but other systemic and topical agents may also be a cause. A case of a 56-year old Korean male was reported with GFDE following application of piroxicam plaster [3]. The patient had similar reactions following a piroxicam injection 3 years before, as well as to topical application of a piroxicam cream. It is unclear why he would repeatedly use piroxicam following two adverse reactions to the drug [3].

The clinical features are usually of well-defined, annular plaques [1–3], with darker centres and paler margins. Our case had annular, ring-like lesions with central clearing. This may perhaps be because of the fairly chronic nature of his disorder.

A case series suggested that fixed drug eruptions accounted for 8.4% of all adverse drug reactions [4], 80.6% of cases were due to antimicrobials, with 20.8% due to non-steroidal anti-inflammatory drugs. Systemic administration was the route in all cases. Interestingly, 66.7% of cases had a prior history of fixed drug eruption [4].

Our case had no history of prior drug intake although, in his line of work, he may not have paid attention to occasional use of systemic or topical agents (for pain relief) and therefore failed to report these even during history taking.

Intradermal CD8+ T-cells are implicated in the pathogenesis of fixed drug reactions [5], leading to epidermal injury possibly via IFN-gamma production [5].

The patient failed to respond to traditional topical and systemic therapies, but responded to homeopathic *Nux vomica* at M potency, given weekly, over a 6-week period and remains in remission (Fig. 23.3a, b).

This is a rare presentation of a non-bullous GFDE mimicking a figurate erythema.

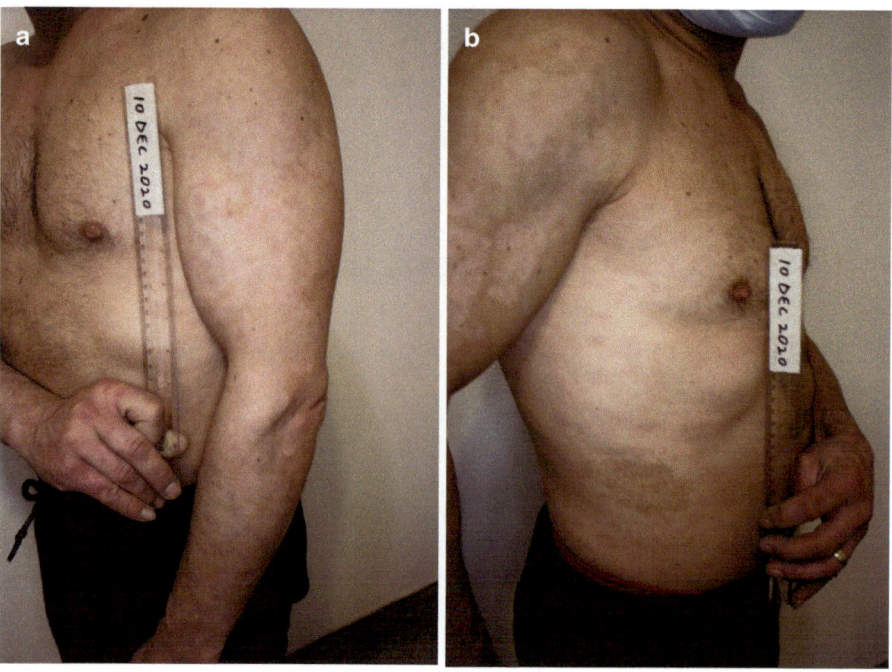

Fig. 23.3 (**a, b**) Lesions in remission, with only residual postinflammatory leukoderma in some areas

Key Points
- Fixed drug eruptions may be localised or generalised
- Antimicrobials are the overwhelming cause of fixed drug eruption
- Occasionally, topical agents may cause GFDE
- Bullous GFDE are more common than the non-bullous variety.
- Rarely, GFDE may mimic a figurate erythema.

References

1. Kornmehl H, Gorouhi F, Konia T, Fung MA, Tartar DM. Generalized fixed drug eruption to piperacillin/tazobactam and review of literature. Dermatol Online J. 2018;24(4):13030/qt8cr714g5.
2. Iliyas M, Ram Subba Reddy M, Devi U. Ciprofloxacin-induced generalised non-bullous fixed drug eruption. BMJ Case Rep. 2018.;2018:bcr2018224858; https://doi.org/10.1136/bcr-2018-224858.
3. Rho YK, Yoo KH, Kim BJ, Kim MN, Song KY. A case of generalized fixed drug eruption due to a piroxicam plaster. Clin Exp Dermatol. 2010;35(2):204–5. https://doi.org/10.1111/j.1365-2230.2009.03394.x.
4. Jhaj R, Chaudhary D, Asati D, Sadasivam B. Fixed-drug eruptions: what can we learn from a case series? Indian J Dermatol. 2018;63(4):332–7. https://doi.org/10.4103/ijd.IJD_481_17.
5. Shiohara T, Mizukawa Y. Fixed drug eruption: a disease mediated by self-inflicted responses of intraepidermal T cells. Eur J Dermatol. 2007;17(3):201–8. https://doi.org/10.1684/ejd.2007.0149.

Chapter 24
Numerous Nodules on the Forehead

Qu Qi and Xing-Hua Gao

A 40-year-old male patient presented to The First Hospital of China Medical University outpatient with a complaint of swelling nodules on the eyebrow that had lasted for 2 years. He claimed that his forehead and neck had kept getting small skin-color bumps since 2018, the skin lesions were mainly painless masses, with occasional severe itching. In the past 2 years, the course of the disease was slowly progressive. Through consultation, we get information that the man had no other chronic disease but had suffered from eczema attacks periodically for 3 years. Physical examination revealed that the patient had many small skin-color nodules on the forehead and diffuse swelling between the eyebrows (Fig. 24.1a, b).

Based on the Case Description and the Photograph, What Is Your Diagnosis?

1. Kimura's disease
2. Angiolymphoid hyperplasia with eosinophilia (ALHE)
3. Eosinophilic granuloma
4. Lymphoma

The results of laboratory examination were obtained, which showed increased peripheral blood eosinophil count of 0.63×10^9/L (normal range: $0.02–0.52^9$/L) and serum IgE level in serum of 817 IU/mL (normal range: <0–100 IU/mL) significantly increased. The results of other laboratory tests were all in normal ranges.

Q. Qi · X.-H. Gao (✉)
Department of Dermatology, The First Hospital of China Medical University,
Shenyang, China

T. M. Lotti et al. (eds.), *Clinical Cases in Facial Erythema*, Clinical Cases in Dermatology, https://doi.org/10.1007/978-3-031-05996-4_24

Fig. 24.1 Clinical manifestation of the patient. (**a**) swelling nodule over the eyebrow arch; (**b**) numerous small skin-color nodules on the forehead and diffuse swelling between the eyebrows

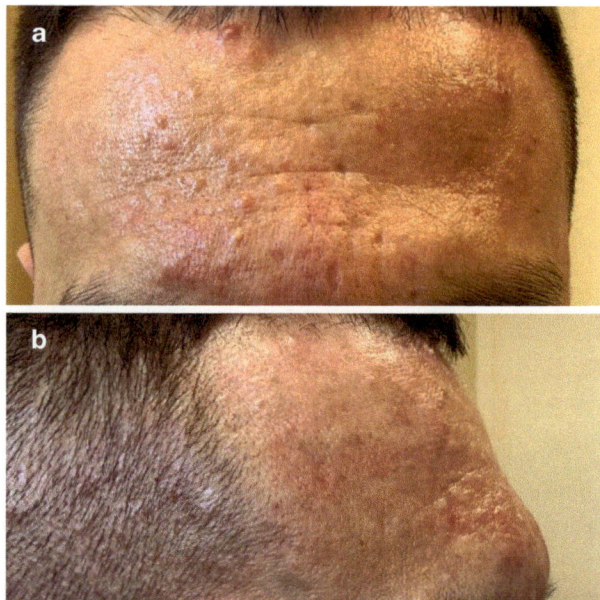

Biopsy report demonstrated there were no special changes in the epidermis. The lesions were mainly in the dermis and subcutaneous tissues. There were significant lymphoid follicle formation with actively hyperplastic germinal centers. There were inflammatory cells, especially obvious eosinophils infiltration with formation of eosinophilic microabscesses, small blood vessel dilitation and fibrous tissue proliferation.

Diagnosis

Kimura's disease.

Discussion

Kimura's disease is a rare chronic benign inflammatory condition with unknown etiology, which is mainly observed in young men of Asian (Chinese and Japanese) between 20 and 40 years of age. It involves subcutaneous single or multiple nodules without pain in head and neck region, characterized by the formation of multiple lymphoid follicles with prominent germinal centers, many of which are infiltrated by eosinophils. It is easy to form eosinophilic microabscesses, which may be accompanied with different degrees of fibrosis and angiogenesis. The lesions are deeply seated and usual presentation are painlessly enlarged lymph nodes with submandibular and parotid gland involvement, however, other organs and systems are rarely involed. The eyelid, eye, oral cavity, chest and extremities may also be involved in rare cases. Most reported cases are typically associated with elevated serum IgE level and peripheral blood eosinophil counts. Some Kimura's disease patients are accompanied with asthma, allergic rhinitis, eczema and ulcerative colitis and so on [1].

ALHE is reported to mimic Kimura's disease, but we can distinguish these two diseases by special characteristics. Firstly, in contrast to Kimura's disease, ALHE is more common in middle-aged women in the Westen nations. The skin lesions are also benign angiomatous nodules or plaques, which occur often in clusters and locate in the head-neck region, especially around the ears, forehead and scalp. It can occur asymptomatically or with pain, itching and pulsation. Secondly, ALHE skin lesions have pathological characteristics of dermal and subcutaneous localized, well-defined, lobulated vascular hyperplasia, vascular endothelial cells swelling and proliferating protrution to the lumen, accompanied by diffuse eosinophil and lymphocyte infiltration. Compared with Kimura's disease, follicles with active germinal centers and eosinophilic abscesses are rarely seen. Moreover, peripheral blood eosinophil counts and serum IgE levels are mostly normal in patients with ALHE [2].

Eosinophilic granuloma pathological changes are also characterized by cellular hyperplasia, but it is more commonly appear in children. The lesions mainly involve bone, and extra-osseous tissues such as lymph nodes, skin and lungs are rarely observed. Although Kimura's disease also has rare cases involving bone tissue, the two can be distinguished by pathological examination. The main component of eosinophilic granuloma lesions is the lamella hyperplasia of Langerhans cells, which are scattered among a large number of eosinophils, neutrophils and lymphocytes. Electron microscopy shows that the cytoplasm of Langerhans cells contains Birbeck granules. In the late stage of the disease, eosinophils number decreases gradually, and the proliferation of fibrous tissue eventually leads to fibrosis of the lesion [3].

Lymphoma is worth mentioning in the differential diagnosis of this case because it has similar clinical manifestation and histological changes with Kimura's disease. Lymphoma is a group of heterogeneous neoplastic diseases that can occur in any part of the body. Lymph nodes, tonsils, spleen and bone marrow are most easily affected. Painless, progressive lymphadenopathy and local masses are its characteristic clinical manifestations, which may be accompanied by symptoms of compression of other organs. Generally speaking, lymphoma is a systemic disease that is accompanied by systemic symptoms such as fever, night sweats, weight loss and itching. When the lesion invades the extranodal tissues, such as the skin, a series of non-specific skin manifestations may appear. For example, skin damage, erythema, nodules, papules, etc. Lymphomas are divided into two categories according to histopathological characteristics: Hodgkin's lymphoma and non-Hodgkin's lymphoma. The pathological manifestations vary according to the type of lymphoma. The diagnosis of lymphoma and the determination of the classification and stage need to rely on pathological biopsy of the lymph node or the cumulative location of the lesion [4].

The patient's medical history, clinical picture, the pathological and laboratory examinations confirmed the diagnosis of Kimura's disease.

The patient was previously treated with thalidomide for 2–3 months but he felt the therapy was no effect. The patient was instructed to take oral minocycline capsules 50 mg twice a day and topical halometasone cream. It should be noted that halometasone cream should not be used for more than 3 weeks. The doctors took photo records of the patient's skin lesions to help follow-up comparative observations.

Key Points

- Kimura's disease is a rare benign lymphoproliferative disease without definite etiology.
- Kimura's disease usually occurs in the head, neck and extremities, and regional lymph nodes are affected frequently.
- Auxiliary examinations that strongly elevated serum IgE levels and blood eosinophil count prompt Kimura's disease. However, the final diagnosis depends on pathological features.

References

Gurram P, et al. Kimura's disease - an e[x]clusive condition. Ann Maxillofac Surg. 2019;9(1):183–7.

Theofilou NE, et al. Angiolymphoid hyperplasia with eosinophilia located on the forehead: a possible association with oral contraceptive use? Dermatopathology(Basel). 2019;6(4):225–30.

Bajracharya B, et al. Eosinophilic granuloma of mandible: a diagnostic challenge. Kathmandu Univ Med J (KUMJ). 2018;16(62):201–3.

Kempf W, et al. Cutaneous lymphomas-An update 2019. Hematol Oncol. 2019;37(1):43–7.

Chapter 25
One Patient with Facial Tan Patches

Ya-Ning Jiao, Nan Yu, Xin-Hong Ge, Li Xia, Yuan-Yuan Shang, and Ke-Xin Li

A 54-year-old woman presented with multiple tan patches on her face for 20 years. Based on the case description and photos (Fig. 25.1), what is your diagnosis?

1. Lichen planus
2. Verruca plana

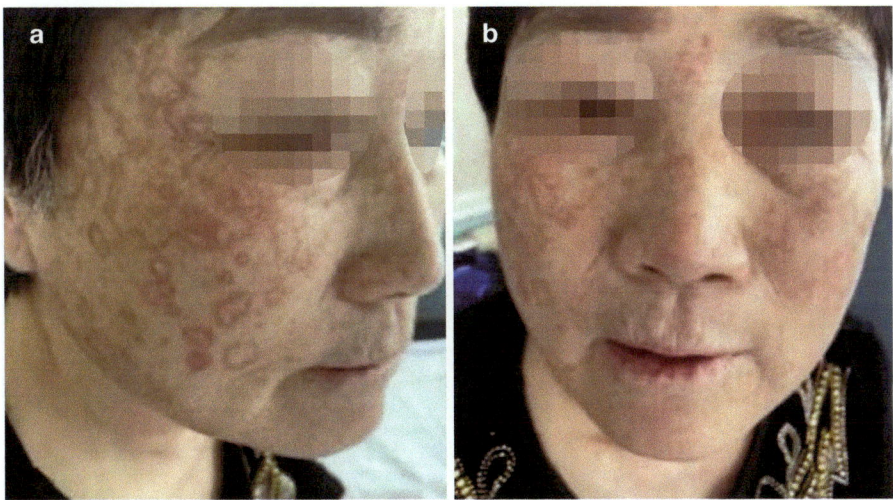

Fig. 25.1 Clinical manifestation of the patient. (**a**) lateral lesions of the face; (**b**) facial lesions on the front

Y.-N. Jiao · N. Yu (✉) · X.-H. Ge · L. Xia · Y.-Y. Shang · K.-X. Li
Department of Dermatology, Affiliated Hospital of Ningxia Medical University,
Yinchuan, China

T. M. Lotti et al. (eds.), *Clinical Cases in Facial Erythema*, Clinical Cases in
Dermatology, https://doi.org/10.1007/978-3-031-05996-4_25

3. Actinic keratosis
4. Verrucous epidermal nevus
5. Granuloma annulare perforans
6. Annular elastolytic granuloma
7. Creeping penetrating elastosis

Medical History

Twenty years ago, several scattered reddish rashes appeared on the right side of the face without obvious inducement, without subjective symptoms, and no attention was paid to them. Later, the rashes progressively increased, gradually involving the left side of the face, and gradually expanded to form annular, geographic and irregular well-defined patches, and the rashes significantly increased in the past 1 year. His mother and one sister had similar rashes on the face. Skin biopsy showed corns lamina (cell column composed of dyskeratotic cells) in the stratum corneum, reduced granular layer below it, cytoplasmic eosinophilic and nuclear hyperchromatic dyskeratotic cells in the spinous cell layer, and lymphocyte infiltration around superficial dermal vessels (Fig. 25.2).

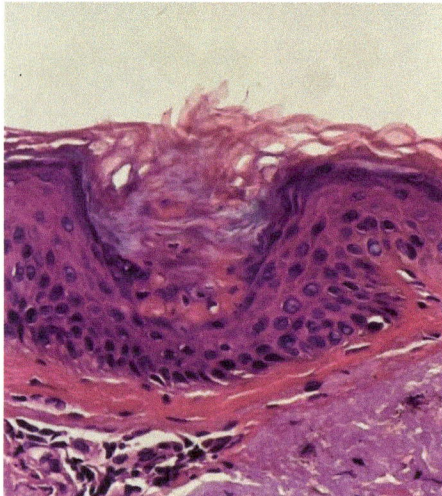 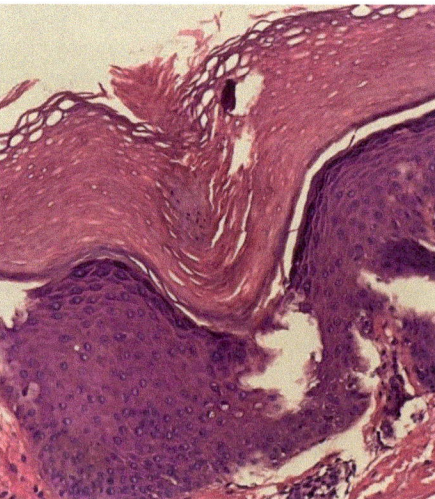

Fig. 25.2 Skin biopsy showed corns lamina (cell column composed of dyskeratotic cells) in the stratum corneum, reduced granular layer below it, cytoplasmic eosinophilic and nuclear hyperchromatic dyskeratotic cells in the spinous cell layer, and lymphocyte infiltration around superficial dermal vessels.(HE×40)

Diagnosis

Porokeratosis.

Discussion

Porokeratosis (PK) was first named by Mibelli in 1983 [1]. Is a Uncommon hereditary chronic parakeratotic dermatosis, autosomal dominant, with long-range familial aggregation, i.e. Its clinical features are mainly keratinizing plaques with dike or verrucous elevation at the margin and mild atrophy in the center, which typically present histopathologically Corns in the epidermis Lamellae [2]. Disease of complex and diverse etiology and pathogenesis [3]. At present, genetic factors, ultraviolet light, trauma, immunosuppression, transplant patients, infectious factors and malignant tumors may be related to PK pathogenesis [4].

The disease is rare in males, most of them are in early childhood, a few begin in adulthood, and generally have no subjective symptoms. The lesions are initially small keratinizing papules that slowly expand to form annular, ground pattern, creeping or irregular well-defined patches with dike and grooved keratinous elevations at the edges, gray or brown, dry and smooth skin or mild atrophy in the central part, lack vellus hair, and large and fine keratinous plugs at the pinpoint can be found in the pores between them. The disease is good in the extremities, face, neck, shoulder and back and vulva, but also involving the scalp and oral cavity, different parts of the clinical manifestations vary. Lesions tend to persist and progress slowly and irregularly. The clinical classics are plaque type, and there are some special types, such as superficial disseminated type, unilateral linear type, disseminated superficial actinic porokeratosis, marked hyperkeratosis type, inflammatory keratosis type, generalized palmar and metatarsal type, punctate porokeratosis, papular type, verrucous plaque type, and mixed type.

At present, there is no specific effect in the treatment of this disease and standard of treatment, i.e. Localized lesions can be treated with carbon dioxide laser, electrocautery, liquid nitrogen cryotherapy, or surgical resection. External 0 with 10% salicylic acid ointment or 0.05–0.1% tretinoin ointment may also be considered 5-Fluorouracil Encapsulate. In severe cases, oral vitamin A derivative therapy may be considered. Appropriate oral hydroxychloroquine may be given to patients suspected of being related to sunlight exposure. However, various treatments have limited efficacy and cannot limit recurrence.

It is worth noting that porokeratosis is prone to malignant transformation into squamous cell carcinoma, Bowen's disease, and basal cell carcinoma [5, 6]. It often occurs in classic plaque type and current status porokeratosis large, isolated long-term skin lesions, so close follow-up should be performed, the skin lesions of suspicious lesions should be surgically removed as early as possible, genetic counseling is required before marriage and childbearing by family members, and chromosomal examination is conditionally required.

Key Points
- Porokeratosis It is an autosomal dominant genodermatosis.
- The clinical features are mainly keratinizing plaques with dike or verrucous elevation at the margin and mild central atrophy, which typically present histopathologicallyCorns in the epidermis Lamellae.
- Typical histopathological findings are Corns in the epidermis Lamellae.

References

1. Joshi R, Minni K. Genitogluteal porokeratosis: a clini- cal review [J]. Clin Cosmet Investig Dermatol. 2018;11:219–29.
2. Xu YY, Fu XA, Yang BQ, et al. A novel MVK gene mutation in a Chinese patient with disseminated actinic superficial poro- keratosis [J]. Dermatologica Sinica. 2015;33(1):45–6.
3. Kanitakis J, Euvrard S, Faure M, et al. Porokeratosis and immunosuppression [J]. Eur J Dermatol. 1998;8(7):459–65.
4. Mori T, Yamamoto T. Genital porokeratosis with amyloid mimicking deposition extrammary Paget disease [J]. Clin Exp Dermatol. 2017;42(3):336–8.
5. Sertznig P, vonFelbert V, Megahed M. Porokeratosis: present concepts [J]. J Eur Acad Dermatol Venereol. 2012;26(4):404–12.
6. Ahmed A, Hivnor C. A case of genital porokeratosis and review of literature [J]. Indian J Dermatol. 2015;60(2):217.

Chapter 26
Red Face in a 57-Year-Old Patient with Pulmonary Cancer

Selami Aykut Temiz and Recep Dursun

A 57-year-old male patient was referred from the medical oncology department to our dermatology outpatient clinic due to diffuse redness and burning on the face. In the dermatological examination, there were pustules and crusts as well as wide-spread redness on the face (Figs. 26.1 and 26.2). It was learned that the lesions on the patient's face developed within a week. In his medical history, it was learned that the patient had been treated for stage 4 pulmonary squamous cell cancer for 3

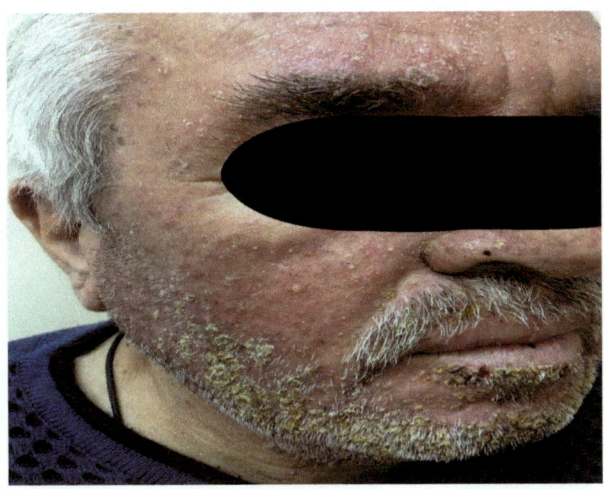

Fig. 26.1 Pustules and crusts as well as widespread redness on the face

S. A. Temiz (✉) · R. Dursun
Department of Dermatology, Necmettin Erbakan University Meram School of Medicine, Konya, Turkey

T. M. Lotti et al. (eds.), *Clinical Cases in Facial Erythema*, Clinical Cases in Dermatology, https://doi.org/10.1007/978-3-031-05996-4_26

Fig. 26.2 The patient with typical red face

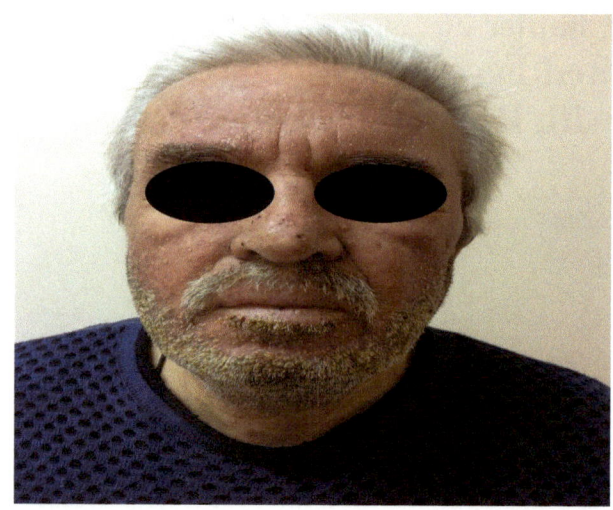

Fig. 26.3 Demodex parasites (Demodex folliculorum and Demodex brevis) in superficial skin surface biopsy from the face

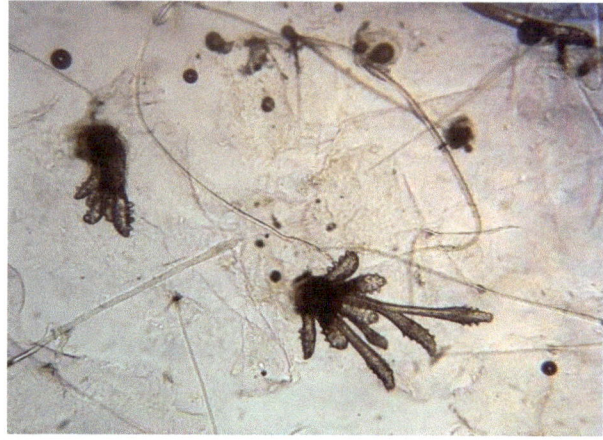

months. The patient was receiving cisplatin and gemcitabine chemotherapy for pulmonary cancer. It was learned from the history of the patient that he was diagnosed with type 2 diabetes mellitus about 10 years ago. The patient was using regular insulin therapy for diabetes mellitus. The superficial skin surface biopsy image made on the patient's face is shown in Fig. 26.3.

Based on the case description and the photos, what is your diagnosis?

1. Papulo-pustular drug reaction
2. Papulo-pustular rosacea
3. Crusted demodicosis
4. Seborrheic dermatitis

Diagnosis

Crusted Demodicosis

The diagnosis of drug eruption was primarily considered due to the short history of the patient's lesions and his history of chemotherapeutic drug use. However, when superficial skin surface biopsy was performed for the differential diagnosis of demodicosis, it was found that there were 42 demodex parasites per cm². As a result of clinical examinations and superficial skin surface biopsy, the patient was diagnosed with crusted demodicosis. The lesions regressed in a short time with antiparasitic therapy.

Discussion

Demodex mites are compulsory commensals that spend all of their life stages in pilosebaceous units, both in animals and humans. D. folliculorum and D. brevis are the most common demodex species in humans, and these demodex mites are also the most common ectoparasites in humans [1]. Demodex parasites can also be found in healthy adults (<5/cm²). Increase in the number of demodex mites, presence of clinical symptoms and improvement with acaricidal treatment are considered as demodicosis [2]. Demodicosis and rosacea can cause similar clinically lesions. However, it may help distinguish some differences in clinical and medical history. In demodicosis, the lesions are superficial and the squames are follicular. Lesions start suddenly and progress rapidly. There is no history of typical flushing, persistent erythema, photosensitivity and telangiectasia like rosacea, and the amount of mites is abundant [1]. In our case, a diagnosis of demodicosis was considered with typical clinical symptoms and the presence of demodex mites, and acaricidal treatment was given. The regression of the lesions with acaricidal treatment made our diagnosis definite.

Although demodex parasites can be found in people of all ages, it is known that positivity rates increase in proportion to the sebum rate in the skin due to age [3]. In addition to the number of demodex mites, environmental and immunological factors are effective in the development of demodicosis. In the literature, it is thought that demodicosis causes more severe clinical conditions in immunocompromised patients [4, 5]. In a study of patients with chronic diseases, it was found that demodicosis was more common in patients with a history of diabetes, hypertension, chronic renal failure, and cancer than in the control group [6]. It has been found that demodicosis is more common in cancer patients than in the normal population. This condition is thought to be possibly due to cancer and immunosuppression by chemotherapy [7]. It was thought that demodicosis in our case caused widespread red face and its crusted course was related to the diabetes and cancer history of our case. It should definitely be considered in demodicosis in addition to drug eruptions and carcinoid syndrome, especially in patients receiving cancer treatment, in the rapidly developing and progressing red face clinic.

Key Points
- Increase in the number of demodex mites ($>5/cm^2$), presence of clinical symptoms and improvement with acaricidal treatment are considered as demodicosis
- Demodicosis may cause more severe clinical conditions in immunocompromised patients (e.g. primary immunodeficiency, cancer, etc.) and patients with chronic disease (e.g. diabetes, hypertension, chronic renal failure)
- It should definitely be considered in demodicosis in addition to drug eruptions and carcinoid syndrome, especially in patients receiving cancer treatment, in the rapidly developing and progressing red face

References

1. Forton F, De Maertelaer V. Two consecutive standardized skin surface biopsies: an improved sampling method to evaluate demodex density as a diagnostic tool for rosacea and demodicosis. Acta Derm Venereol. 2017;97(2):242–8.
2. Dursun R, Durmaz K, Oltulu P, Ataseven A. Demodex positive discoid lupus erythematosus: is it a separate entity or an overlap syndrome? Dermatol Ther. 2020;33:e13394.
3. Akilov OE, Mumcuoglu KY. Immune response in demodicosis. J Eur Acad Dermatol Venereol. 2004;18(4):440–4.
4. Chovatiya RJ, Colegio OR. Demodicosis in renal transplant recipients. Am J Transplant. 2016;16(2):712–6.
5. Caccavale S, Di Mattia D, Ruocco E. Loco-regional immune default: the immunocompromised district in human and comparative dermatology. Clin Dermatol. 2016;34(5):654–7.
6. Cengiz ZT, Ozkol HU, Beyhan YE, Ozturk M, Yilmaz H. Evaluation of some chronical diseases in etiopathogenesis of demodicosis. Dermatol Sin. 2017;35(4):173–6.
7. Van Atteveld JE, Graaf MD, Grotel MV, van den Heuvel-Eibrink MM. Demodicosis in pediatric cancer. J Pediatr Hematol Oncol. 2017;39(5):402–6.

Chapter 27
Red Facial Patches on the Forehead

Uwe Wollina

A 47-year-old man presented with two red patches on his forehead. He reported no subjective symptoms like burning or itch. He did not remember any trauma. Their consistency was soft (Figs. 27.1 and 27.2).

Based upon history and clinical appearance, what is your diagnosis?

1. Hematoma.
2. Fixed drug eruption (FDA).
3. Angiosarcoma.
4. Spider hemangioma.
5. Tufted angioma.

Fig. 27.1 Two red patches on the forehead

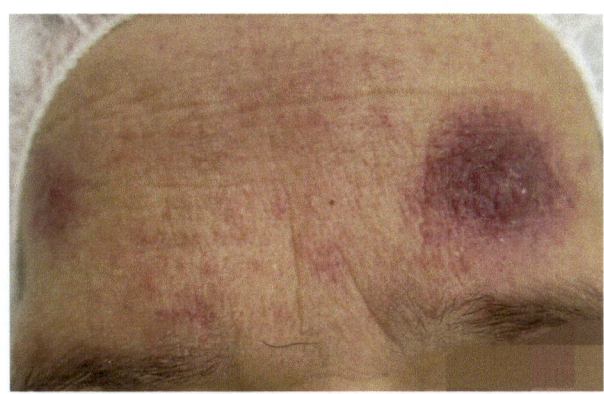

U. Wollina (✉)
Department of Dermatology and Allergology, Städtisches Klinikum Dresden, Academic Teaching Hospital of the Technical University of Dresden, Dresden, Germany
e-mail: Uwe.Wollina@klinikum-dresden.de

Fig. 27.2 Detail with central slightly elevated plaque and scaling

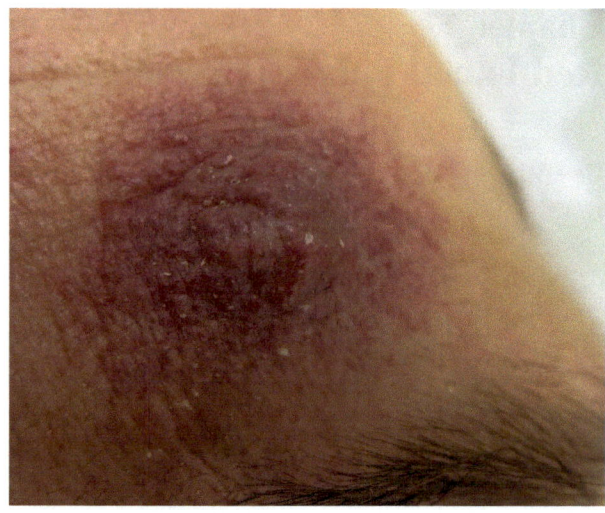

Diagnosis Spider hemangioma in chronic alcoholism with liver cirrhosis.

On examination, we observed two erythematous lesions, about 3–4 cm in diameter, with a central slightly elevated soft plaque and both sides of the forehead. On his cheeks and trunk numerous classical spider nevi were seen. He also presented palmar erythema and gynecomastia.

Laboratory investigations: Erythrocyte count 3.77 Tpt/l (normal range 4.6–6.2), hemoglobin 8.4 mmol/l (8.6–12.1), thrombocytes 49.0 Gpt/l (120–340), Quick 50.0% (70–130), fibrinogen 1.28 g/l (2.0–5.0), activated prothrombin time 35.5 s (26–35), gamma-glutamyl transferase 3.97 μkat/l (<1.10).

Esophagoscopy demonstrated esophageal varices.

Skin biopsy from a lesion of the forehead: Telangiectatic capillaries.

Discussion

Chronic alcoholism can lead to cirrhosis, resulting in end-stage liver disease. Defective synthesis of clotting factors due to compromised hepatic synthesis may leads to bleeding disorders. Cutaneous changes can be of significant diagnostic value in alcoholism-associated cirrhosis. Spider nevi and larger angiomas as in our case, palmar erythema, hypotrichosis and Dupuytren's contracture are commonly seen. Acquired zinc deficiency can cause eczematous lesions with periorificial manifestations. Pellagra and pellagroid-like changes may occur. Most characteristic lesions of alcoholic cirrhosis include paper money skin and Dupuytren's contracture. These skin changes also help in diagnosis and staging of liver cirrhosis [1, 2].

Specific vascular lesions have to be excluded by histopathology such as rare adult Kasabach-Merritt phenomenon [3], kaposiform hemangioendothelioma and tufted angioma [4], unilateral nevoid telangiectasia [1], and angiosarcoma [5].

Increased amounts of circulating vascular endothelial growth factor have been detected in chronic liver disease, what might be at least in part responsible for cutaneous vascular lesions [6].

Key Points
- Spider nevi and plaque-like telangiectatic lesions are a hallmark of alcohol-induced liver cirrhosis.
- Cutaneous lesions such as paper money skin may be a diagnostic clue.
- Atypical vascular lesions need histologic confirmation to exclude malignancies.

References

1. Capron JP, Kantor G, Dupas JL, Degott C, Locquet MC. Unilateral nevoid telangiectasia and chronic liver disease. Report of a case and review of the literature. Am J Gastroenterol. 1981;76(1):47–51.
2. Dogra S, Jindal R. Cutaneous manifestations of common liver diseases. J Clin Exp Hepatol. 2011;1(3):177–84.
3. Fernandez AP, Wolfson A, Ahn E, Maldonad JC, Alonso-Llamazares J. Kasabach-Merritt phenomenon in an adult man with a tufted angioma and cirrhosis responding to radiation, bevacizumab, and prednisone. Int J Dermatol. 2014;53(9):1165–76.
4. Chu CY, Hsiao CH, Chiu HC. Transformation between kaposiform hemangioendothelioma and tufted angioma. Dermatology. 2003;206(4):334–7.
5. Wollina U. Angiosarcoma: an immunogenic tumour. Br J Dermatol. 2018;179(2):257–8.
6. Makhlouf MM, Awad A, Zakhari MM, Fouad M, Saleh WA. Vascular endothelial growth factor level in chronic liver diseases. J Egypt Soc Parasitol. 2002;32(3):907–21.

Chapter 28
Red-Purple Plaque on the Right Side of the Neck

Filippo Viviani, Alba Guglielmo, Carlotta Baraldi, Federica Filippi, Alessandro Pileri, and Federico Bardazzi

Case Presentation

A 69-year-old woman came to the Author's attention with a tender, red-purple plaque on the right side of the neck. The lesion was asymptomatic and had raised, swollen margins. It had appeared 6 weeks before and had gradually enlarged, subsequently also affecting the chest area. On suspicion of erysipelas, the patient had been treated with penicillin and ceftriaxone, with no improvement. She reported the onset of dyspepsia in the previous months but denied any fever or other systemic symptoms. Her medical history included hypertension, type 2 diabetes and chronic gastritis. General laboratory tests showed no alterations and, at physical examination, we found axillary and cervical lymphadenopathy (Figs. 28.1, 28.2 and 28.3).

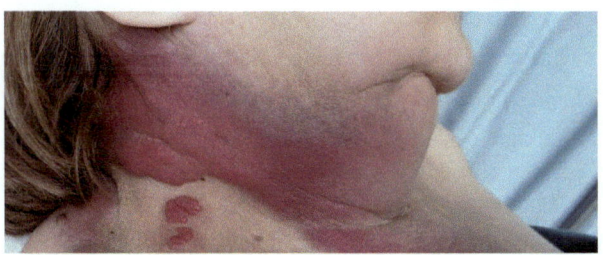

Fig. 28.1 Tender, red-purple plaque on the right side of the neck

F. Viviani · A. Guglielmo · C. Baraldi · F. Filippi · A. Pileri (✉) · F. Bardazzi
Dermatology -IRCCS Policlinico di Sant'Orsola, Department of Experimental, Diagnostic and Specialty Medicine (DIMES), Alma Mater Studiorum University of Bologna, Bologna, Italy
e-mail: filippo.viviani3@studio.unibo.it; alessandro.pileri2@unibo.it; federico.bardazzi@aosp.bo.it

© The Author(s), under exclusive license to Springer Nature Switzerland AG 2022
T. M. Lotti et al. (eds.), *Clinical Cases in Facial Erythema*, Clinical Cases in Dermatology, https://doi.org/10.1007/978-3-031-05996-4_28

Fig. 28.2 Tender, red-purple plaque on the chest and neck

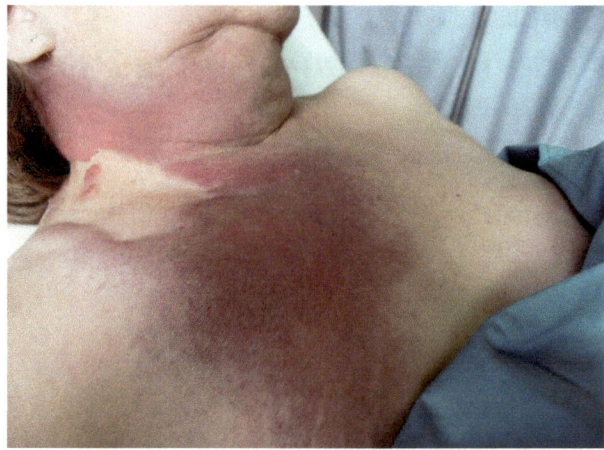

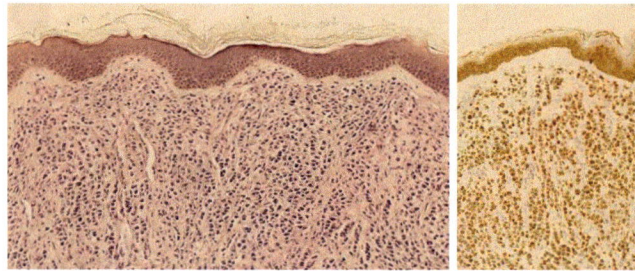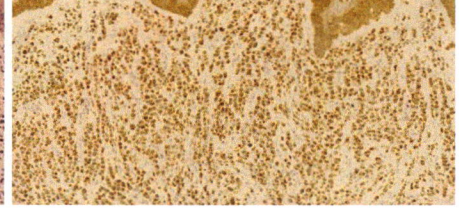

Fig. 28.3 Histopathological and immunohistochemical study on a punch biopsy showed a dense dermal deposition of plasmacytoid cells positive for Cytokeratin MNF 116 and E-cadherin indicated a cutaneous localization of adenocarcinoma

Based upon the history and clinical appearance, what is your diagnosis?

1. Cellulitis
2. Cutaneous T-cell lymphoma
3. Erysipelas carcinomatosum
4. Angiosarcoma

Diagnosis Gastric adenocarcinoma-derived erysipelas earcinomatosum.

Discussion

Histopathological and immunohistochemical study on a punch biopsy showed a dense dermal deposition of plasmacytoid cells positive for Cytokeratin MNF 116 and E-cadherin indicated a cutaneous localization of adenocarcinoma. A subsequent gastroscopy diagnosed a gastric adenocarcinoma. Therefore, a diagnosis of erysipelas earcinomatosum (EC, also known as inflammatory carcinoma) was made. This condition resembles an erysipelas (a plaque of thickened, red skin with raised margins), and is caused by a diffuse spreading of tumor cells within the lymphatic vessels [1]. EC is most commonly found in the chest area but may uncommonly involve the head and neck region. Other possible differential diagnoses include angiosarcoma, cutaneous T-cell lymphoma, radiation dermatitis and herpes zoster [2]. Usually, EC is observed in association with breast cancer and cutaneous melanoma, but other adenocarcinomas, such as thyroid, parotid gland, stomach, pancreas, larynx, prostate, carcinomas, can determine this condition [3]. It is still unclear why some cutaneous metastases present with a more inflammatory appearance: both the inflammatory properties of specific malignancies and a heterogeneity in the host response to the spread of the tumor may play a role [4]. The diagnosis can be difficult and EC should be suspected when monolateral, asymptomatic erysipelas-like lesions in the chest area, unassociated with fever, are unresponsive to antibiotic therapy [2]. However, histopathology and immunohistochemistry play a fundamental role in the diagnostic process. The management of this skin condition follows that of the primary tumor, nonetheless the prognosis is often poor.

Key Points
- Erysipelas earcinomatosum presents as a plaque of thickened, red skin with raised margins, and is caused by a diffuse spreading of tumor cells within the lymphatic vessels.
- Usually, it is observed in association with breast cancer but also urogenital and gastrointestinal carcinomas can determine this condition.
- Erysipelas earcinomatosum should be suspected when monolateral, asymptomatic erysipelas-like lesions, unassociated with fever, are unresponsive to antibiotic therapy.
- Histopathology and immunohistochemistry play a fundamental role in the diagnostic process.

References

1. Müller CSL, Pföhler C, Reichrath J, Tilgen W. Erysipelas carcinomatosum der Abdominalhaut: "Erstmanifestation" eines Siegelringzellkarzinoms des Magens. Hautarzt. 2008;59(12):992–4. https://doi.org/10.1007/s00105-008-1541-z.
2. Hariry H, Abeler T, Melnik B, Vakilzadeh F. Erysipelas carcinomatosum in tubular adenocarcinoma of the stomach. Hautarzt Z Dermatol Venerol Verwandte Geb. 2000;51(12):950–2. https://doi.org/10.1007/s001050051246.
3. Goldust M, Heinz J, Gupta M, Grabbe S. Merkel cell carcinoma-derived Erysipelas carcinomatosum. Dermatol Ther. 2020;33(3):e13287. https://doi.org/10.1111/dth.13287.
4. Cox SE, Cruz PD. A spectrum of inflammatory metastasis to skin via lymphatics: three cases of carcinoma erysipeloides. J Am Acad Dermatol. 1994;30(2):304–7. https://doi.org/10.1016/S0190-9622(94)70028-1.

Chapter 29
Ulcero-Crusted Lesions of the Face

Diego Abbenante, Miriam Anna Carpanese, Michelangelo La Placa, and Federico Bardazzi

A 65-year-old previously healthy man presented to our clinic with multiple skin lesions on the left side of the face. He reported that the lesions had appeared 6 days before as small fluid-filled vesicles and their aspect had changed over the days.

He complained of liquid swallowing difficulty and left otalgia (Figs. 29.1 and 29.2).

Based upon the history and clinical appearance, what is your diagnosis?

1. Dermatitis artefacta
2. Trigeminal trophic syndrome
3. Ramsay Hunt syndrome
4. Bullous impetigo

Diagnosis Ramsay Hunt syndrome.

On examination, we observed several crusted lesions on an erythematous base in a linear arrangement from the left ear to the perioral region. Yellow exudation was observed on the surface of the external auditory canal. An otolaryngology consultation excluded a tympanic membrane involvement. Physical examination revealed facial asymmetry consistent with peripheral facial nerve palsy. On the basis of clinical findings, we made the diagnosis of Ramsay Hunt syndrome.

Oral prednisone 25 mg once daily and valaciclovir 1000 mg 3-times/day were started and the patient improved following the treatment.

D. Abbenante · M. A. Carpanese · M. La Placa · F. Bardazzi (✉)
Dermatology Unit, IRCCS Azienda Ospedaliero-Universitaria di Bologna, Bologna, Italy
e-mail: diego.abbenante@studio.unibo.it; michelangelo.laplaca@unibo.it; federico.bardazzi@aosp.bo.it

Fig. 29.1 Ulcero-crusted
lesions in a linear
disposition on the left side
of the face

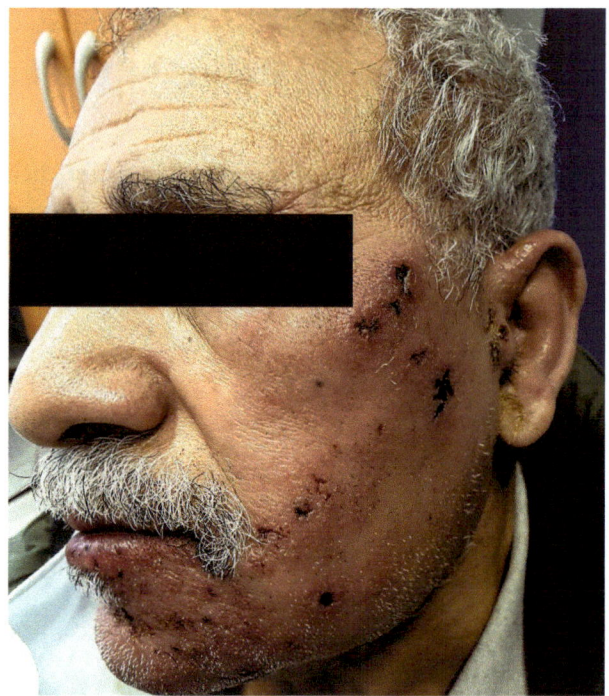

Discussion

Ramsay Hunt syndrome develops due to the reactivation and replication of varicella-zoster virus in the geniculate ganglion of the facial nerve. Classical symptoms include facial palsy, otalgia, and skin lesions that arise along the course of the facial nerve. Dizziness and hearing loss may be present, but less often [1]. Patients typically refer a burning sensation, while dysphagia is reported only in few cases and can be explained by other cranial nerves involvement [2].

Skin signs may appear after the facial neuropathy. Cutaneous lesions begin as red macules and papules that, in the course of 7–10 days, form a vesicular rash that evolve into pustules and crusts.

Ramsay Hunt syndrome is estimated to account for 18% of facial palsies in adults [3]. Even if this syndrome is a self-limiting condition, various complications are possible including bacterial superinfection, residual facial weakness, encephalitis or meningitis.

Combined therapy using oral corticosteroids and oral antiviral agents is commonly used in the treatment of Ramsay Hunt syndrome. Clinical studies show that starting treatment in the first week is correlated with the highest rate of improvement, although treatment started later still has some benefit [4].

Fig. 29.2 Close-up view
of the pinna showing
oozing, crusted lesions

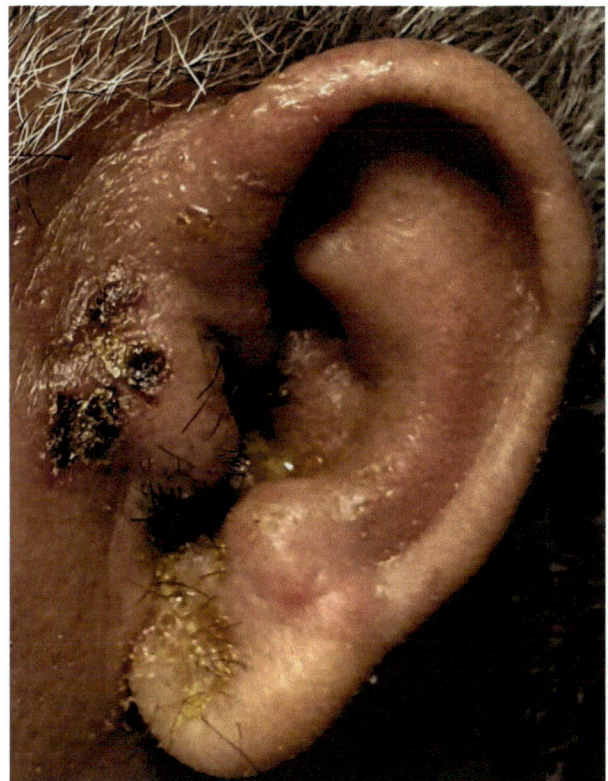

Key Points

- Ramsay Hunt syndrome is a severe presentation of varicella-zoster virus reacti-
  vation in the geniculate ganglion.
- Some patients develop vesicles after facial nerve palsy therefore such cases can
  be misdiagnosed.
- It is important to look for auricular vesicles in all patients with facial nerve palsy.
- Earlier start of treatment is correlated with better outcomes.

References

1. Jeon Y, Lee H. Ramsay Hunt syndrome. J Dent Anesth Pain Med. 2018;18(6):333–7.
2. Shim JH, Park JW, Kwon BS, et al. Dysphagia in Ramsay Hunt's syndrome—a case report.
   Ann Rehabil Med. 2011;35(5):738–41.
3. Gilchrist JM. Seventh cranial neuropathy. Semin Neurol. 2009;29(1):5–13.
4. Ryu EW, Lee HY, Lee SY, Park MS, Yeo SG. Clinical manifestations and prognosis of patients
   with Ramsay Hunt syndrome. Am J Otolaryngol. 2012;33(3):313–8.

Chapter 30
Unilateral Erythema

Monika Fida, Ritjana Mala, and Oljeda Kaçani

Case Report A 46-year-old woman presented in our Dermatology Department with one year history of unilateral facial flushing and sweating affecting only the left side of the face. At the same time the other side remaining pale and dry. These manifestations were provoked by physical exercise during hot weather or emotional stress. Her previous medical history revealed a hospitalization in pulmonary hospital before she presented to our department. Patient had been admitted to the Department of Pneumology for exertion dyspnea and was diagnosed and treated for First Stage Sarcoidosis. Thoracic CT scan had revealed only hilar and paratracheal lymph nodes enlargement. She had no other significant medical history. There was no history of undergoing any surgical procedure. Her family medical history was unremarkable. On physical examination no sweating or flushing was noted at rest. Her vital signs were normal. No pupillary abnormalities including signs of Horner syndrome were observed. A detailed eye examination performed by an ophthalmologist revealed no abnormalities. Laboratory evaluation including complete blood count, ESR, glycemia, renal, hepatic and thyroid function tests were all normal. ANA test was found to be positive (++). During the neurological examination, including cranial nerves exam, motor and sensory systems evaluation, higher mental function, deep tendon reflexes did not result any abnormality. The symptoms (an erythematous flushing and sweating on the left side of her face) were evident after a 30-minutes excessive walking or running in hot weather. These symptoms were alleviated by cold compresses and after stopping the physical activity. During the episode the pupils were equal in size and reacted normally to light. Her vital signs were also normal. A CT scan of the head and neck revealed only bilaterally latero-

M. Fida (✉) · R. Mala · O. Kaçani
Dermatology Department, Faculty of Medicine, University of Medicine of Tirana,
Tirana, Albania
e-mail: monika.fida@fakultetimjekesise.edu.al

© The Author(s), under exclusive license to Springer Nature
Switzerland AG 2022
T. M. Lotti et al. (eds.), *Clinical Cases in Facial Erythema*, Clinical Cases in
Dermatology, https://doi.org/10.1007/978-3-031-05996-4_30

Fig. 30.1 Evident hemifacial erythema just in one side

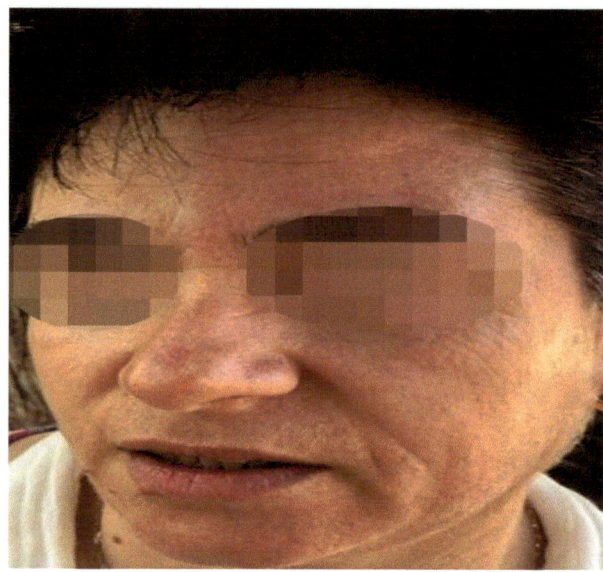

cervical lymph node enlargement of 6 mm without any structural lesion. A Doppler ultrasound of the carotid arteries resulted normal (Fig. 30.1).

Based on the case description and the photograph, what is your diagnosis?
- Horner syndrome (miosis, ptosis and enophthalmos)
- Ross syndrome (tonic pupils, segmental anhidrosis and hyporeflexia)
- Holmes-Adie syndrome (tonic pupil and areflexia)
- Harlequin Syndrome?

Diagnosis

Harlequin syndrome.

Discussions

The diagnosis of Harlequin syndrome was made by excluding other possible diagnosis. Asymmetrical facial sweating and flushing has been named the "Harlequin sign" [1, 2]. Harlequin syndrome is a rare autonomic disorder first described by Lance et Drummond 1988 as a manifestation of unilateral facial flushing and sweating during hot weather or when exercising [1]. It was first thought that the occlusion of an anterior radicular artery during exercise was the pathogenic mechanism to explain the symptoms, but the real origin of this syndrome is a dysfunction of the sympathetic chain. The neural damage of the sympathetic system affects the non-flushing side, and the flushing side of the face (arms and trunk sometimes) is known to be a compensatory over reaction [3].

Is Harlequin sign just a color change? When an acute unilateral color change occurs in a patient's appearance, it should be first considered a neurovascular cause. As such a cause may be immediately life threatening, neurovascular disease should be excluded before other potential causes are considered. According to case reports, unilateral facial flushing can be a sign of acute stroke, possibly due to failure of the autonomic nervous system [4].

Different diagnosis taken in consideration are: Horner syndrome with miosis, ptosis and enophthalmos which may indicate a lesion of the superior cervical ganglion; Ross syndrome with tonic pupils, anhidrosis and hyporeflexia which may indicate a lesion of the postganglionic cholinergic parasympathetic and sympathetic fibers projecting to the iris; Holmes-Adie syndrome with tonic pupil and areflexia which may be due to a damage of the ciliary ganglion or to the post-ganglionic nerves from inflammation, autoimmune processes, tumors, trauma or complications of surgery [5]. Referring our case Holmes-Adie syndrome, Ross syndrome and Horner syndrome were excluded by the ophthalmological and neurological examination performed that showed no such abnormalities.

Idiopathic etiology is frequent in older children and adults, but other possible causes including iatrogenic lesions and malignances should be excluded. There are case reports of Harlequin syndrome due to epidural anesthesia or other procedures in the cervicothoracic region [4]. More alarming conditions such as neoplasm of superior mediastine and apical lung can be behind a Harlequin sign [6, 7]. Other less frequent causes are neurotropic virus infection, autoimmune diseases as multiple sclerosis, syringomyelia [5, 7].

What is important to do in a case with Harlequin sign? The diagnostic process is important for ruling out malignant causes or iatrogenic ones. A thorough physical, neurological, and ophthalmological examination is essential and followed by radiology tests [7].

In our patient the thoracic and cranio-cervical CT scan performed showed no space occupying lesion. The cervical lymph nodes noticed to the CT scan were due to sarcoidosis diagnosed before. Except for examination ANA positivity no other abnormality was found. Reviewing the literature, we found many cases of autoimmune origin for such syndromes [8–10] and concluded of a possible autoimmune origin for the symptoms of our patient. The patient was reassured of the benign nature of this condition. A possible solution such as sympathectomy lateral to the flushing side was suggested to the patient to help relieve the symptoms. Patient did not accept to receive any treatment. We recommended to follow up.

Key Points
- Harlequin syndrome consists on a unilateral facial flushing and sweating triggered by exercise or hot weather.
- CT scan or MRI are important for the differential diagnosis.
- Mostly no treatment is recommended.

References

1. Lance JW, Drummond PD, Gandevia SC, Morris JG. Harlequin syndrome: the sudden onset of unilateral flushing and sweating. J Neurol Neurosurg Psychiatry. 1988;51:635–42.
2. Montigiani, et al. The "Harlequin Sign". Case description and review of the literature. Ann Ital Med Int. 1998;13(3):173–5.
3. Drummond PD. The effect of sympathetic blockade on facial sweating and cutaneous vascular response to painful stimulation of the eye. Brain. 1993;116:233–41.
4. Boling B, Key C. Harlequin syndrome as a complication of epidural anesthesia. Crit Care Nurse. 2014;34(3):57–61.
5. Willaert WI, Scheltinga MR, Steenhuisen SF, Hiel JA. Harlequin syndrome: two new cases and a management proposal. Acta Neurol Belg. 2009;109:214–20.
6. Duddy ME, Baker MR. Harlequin's darker side. N Engl J Med. 2007:357.
7. Butragueno Laiseca L, Vasquez Lopez M, Polo AA. Harlequin syndrome in a paediatric patient: a diagnostic challenge. Neurologia. 2018;33(7):478–80.
8. Pradeep PV, Benede AK, Harshita SS, Jayashree B. Harlequin syndrome in a case of toxic goiter: a rare association. Case Rep Med. 2011;2011:293076.
9. Vasudevan B, Sawhney MPS, Vishal S. Ross syndrome with ANA positivity: a clue to possible autoimmune origin and treatment with intravenous immunoglobulin. IJD. 2010;55:274–6.
10. Karam C. Harlequin syndrome in a patient with putative autoimmune autonomic ganglionopathy. Auton Neurosci. 2016;194:58–9.

Index

A

Acne rosacea
    clinical signs and symptoms, 100
    daily broad-spectrum sunscreen, 101
    differential diagnosis, 100
    electrosurgery, 101
    etiopathogenesis, 100
    management protocols, 101
    symptoms, 100
    topical agents, 100
    treatment modalities, 100
    vascular lasers, 101
Acne vulgaris, 97
Acquired zinc deficiency, 124
Acute myeloid leukemia (AML), 81
ALK-negative anaplastic large cell
        lymphoma, 5, 7
Allergic contact dermatitis, 98
Anaplastic large cell lymphoma, 6
Angioedema, 60
Asymmetrical poikilodematous erythema, 41

B

Beta-lactam antibiotics, 59
Bilateral facial erysipelas, 59
Birbeck granules, 113
Bradykinin, 60

C

Cellulitis, 59, 83
Cervical idiopathic poikiloderma, *see*
        Poikiloderma of Civatte

Cheilitis
    clinical manifestation, 33
    endogenous factors, 34
    exogenous factors, 34
    management, 35
Chronic alcoholism, 124
Cirrhosis, 124
Contact dermatitis, 27, 60
Copper sensitivity, 105
CREST syndrome, 3, 17
Cutaneous angiosarcoma (cAS)
    aetiological factors, 86
    common mutations, 86
    histopathological examination, 87
    NUP160-SCL43A3, 86
    primary AS, 86
    prognosis, 87
    RAAS, 86
    secondary AS, 86
Cutaneous lupus erythematosus (CLE), 11
Cutis verticis gyrata, 7
Cytarabine, 82

D

Dapsone, 83
Demodex folliculorum mites, 10, 12, 95, 96,
        100, 121
Demodicosis, 120–122
Dental sinus
    causes, 22
    CT examination, 20
Dermatofibrosarcoma Protuberans
        (DFSP), 22

Dental sinus (*Cont.*)
    intraepidermal neutrophilic abscesses, 22
    keratoacanthoma (KA), 22
    oral therapy, 22
    physical examination, 20
    pyogenic granuloma, 22
    sporotrichosis, 22
    surgery, 22
Dermatofibrosarcoma Protuberans (DFSP), 22
Dermatological disorders treatment, 64
Dermatomyositis (DM), 12, 59, 101
    amyopathic dermatomyositis, 54
    classic skin manifestations, 54
    clinical investigations, 53
    diagnosis of, 54
    follow up, 54
    histopathology, 54
    pharmacological treatment, 53
    treatment of, 54
Diffuse erythema, 1, 52
Dilated esophagus, 3
Discoid lupus erythematosus (DLE),
        11, 12, 27
Disseminated herpes zoster infection, 91
Drug reaction with eosinophilia and systemic
        manifestations (DRESS)
        syndrome, 102
Dupuytren's contracture, 124
Dyspepsia, 127

E
Eosinophilia angiolymphoid hyperplasia
        (ALHE), 113
Eosinophilic granuloma, 113
Erysipelas
    bilateral facial erysipelas, 59
    causes, 59
    and cellulitis, 59
    complications, 59
    symptoms, 59
    treatment, 59
Erysipelas earcinomatosum (EC), 127
    diagnosis of, 128
    differential diagnoses, 129
    histopathological and
        immunohistochemical study,
        128, 129
    inflammatory appearance, 129
Erythemato-telangiectatic rosacea (ETR), 97
Erythematous reticular patches, 76
Erythromelanosis follicularis faciei et colli
        (EFFC), 42, 43

F
First Stage Sarcoidosis, 135
Fitzpatrick skin type III, 75

G
Gastric adenocarcinoma, 128
Generalised fixed drug eruption (GFDE)
    clinical features, 108
    ingested antibiotics, 107
    systemic and topical agents, 107
Graft-versus-host disease (GVHD), 39
Gram negative folliculitis, 98
Gynecomastia, 124

H
Harlequin syndrome, 136, 137
Heliotrope rash, 52
Hemifacial erythema, 136
Herpes Zoster Duplex Bilateralis
        (HZDB), 71, 72
Herpes Zoster Duplex Unilateralis
        (HZDU), 71
Hodgkin's lymphoma, 113
Holmes-Adie syndrome, 137
Horner syndrome, 135, 137
Human herpesvirus-8 (HHV-8), 87
Hypertrichosis, 66

I
IgG4-related disease, 31
Intraepidermal neutrophilic abscesses, 22

J
Jessner lymphocytic infiltration, 27
Juvenile xanthogranuloma (JXG), 31

K
Kaposi's sarcoma (KS), 87
Keratinizing plaques, 117
Keratoacanthoma (KA), 22
Kimura's disease, 112–114

L
Langerhans cell histiocytosis (LCH), 31
Leprosy
    clinical diagnosis, 48
    clinical features, 47

clinical manifestation, 46, 48
combined chemotherapy, 48
eye involvement, 48
gene location, 48
histopathological examination, 46
laboratory tests, 46
mycobacterium leprae, 47
neurofibromatosis, 48
nodular xanthomas, 48
seborrheic dermatitis, 48
skin lesion characteristics, 47
tumefaciens, 48
Leprosy tumefaciens, 48
Leukocytosis, 5
Lichen myxedematosus (LM)
atypical form, 39
dermatomyositis, 39
diagnosis of, 39
generalized, 38
graft-versus-host disease (GVHD), 39
high-dosed intravenous immunoglobulins
(IVIg), 39
histopathology, 37, 38
laboratory findings, 37
localized variant, 39
physical examination, 37
scleromyxedema, 39
systemic sclerosis, 39
Lichen planus
chronic erosive oral lichen planus, 62
diagnosis, 62
drugs, 62
etiology, 62
immunologic factors, 62
Lupus erythematosus (LE), 17, 101

M
Mycobacterium leprae, 47

N
National Rosacea Society, 100
Neoplastic lymphoid cells, 5
Neuralgia, 70
Neutrophilic eccrine hidradenitis (NEH)
diagnosis, 83
drug-induced cytotoxic effect, 83
drugs, 82
erythematous papules and plaques, 82
Niacinamide-induced flushing, 43
Niacinamide-induced poikilodermatous
erythema, 43

Nodular xanthomas, 48
Non-Hodgkin's lymphoma, 113
Nuclear atypia, 87

O
Odontogenic Cutaneous Sinus Tract, 22
Oral metronidazole, 66
Otalgia, 131

P
Palmar erythema, 124
Papulopustular rosacea (PPR), 95
demodex mites, 97
first line treatment options, 97
microbiological examination, 95
pathophysiology, 97
subtypes, 97
topical permethrin therapy, 96
Parapsoriasis variegate, 43
Periorbital erythema and edema, 81
Photosensitivity, 51
Poikiloderma of Civatte, 42
aetiopathogenesis, 78
clinical feature, 77
depigmenting agents, 78
differential diagnosis, 78
erythemato-telangiectatic type, 77
histopathological findings, 78
incidence, 77
laser and light-based therapies, 78
Riehl's melanosis, 78
symptoms, 77
treatment, 78
Poikiloderma vasculare atrophicans, 43
Poikilodermatous erythema, 42
Polymorphous light eruption (PLE), 9, 12
Porokeratosis (PK), 117
Pyogenic granuloma, 22

R
Radiation-associated angiosarcoma
(RAAS), 86
Ramsay Hunt syndrome
causes, 132
clinical studies, 132
combined therapy, 132
symptoms, 132
Raynaud's phenomenon, 1
Rheumatoid arthritis (RA), 58
Riehl's melanosis, 78

Right inguinal herniorrhaphy, 105
Rosacea, 3, 17
Rosai-Dorfman-Destombes disease (RDD)
   clinical presentation, 30
   diagnosis, 31
   differential diagnosis, 31
   epidemiological and clinical features, 30
   H&E staining studies, 29
   kinase mutations, 30
   morphological features, 31
   surgical excision, 31
   systemic therapies, 31
   treatment, 29, 31

S
Sarcoidosis
   clinical manifestation, 27
   diagnosis, 25
   etiology, 26
   first-line therapy, 27
   histology, 27
Scleroderma, 17
Scleromyxedema, 39
Seborrheic dermatitis, 48
Shawl sign, 52
Sinus histiocytosis with massive
       lymphadenopathy (SHML), *see*
       Rosai-Dorfman-Destombes
       disease (RDD)
Spider nevi, 124
Spongiotic dermatitis, 34
Sporotrichosis, 22
Stage 4 pulmonary squamous cell cancer, 119
Standardized skin surface biopsy (SSSB)
       procedure, 9

Stewart–Treves syndrome, 87
Systemic autoimmune diseases, 58
Systemic inflammatory response syndrome
       (SIRS), 59
Systemic lupus erythematosus, 4, 59
Systemic sclerosis, 3, 39

T
Tacrolimus, 29
Telangiectases, 15–17
Telangiectasia, 1, 64, 66
Topical corticosteroids (TC)
   adverse effects, 65
   misapplication of, 65
   rebound phenomenon, 65, 66
   replacement therapy, 66
   symptoms, 65
Topical steroid damaged skin, 63, 64
Topical steroid damaged/dependent face
       (TSDF), 16, 65, 66
Tzanck smear, 92

U
Ulcero-crusted lesions, 132
Unilateral facial flushing, 137
Unilateral poikilodermatous erythematous
       rash, 41

V
Valacyclovir, 92
Varicella, 91, 92
Varicella-zoster virus (VZV), 91, 92